KU-113-373

Physical signs of sexual abuse in children

ST. ALBANS CITY HOSPITAL

LIBRARY

*A Report of
the Royal College of Physicians*

1991

THE ROYAL COLLEGE OF PHYSICIANS OF LONDON

Royal College of Physicians of London
11 St Andrews Place, London NW1 4LE

Copyright © 1991 Royal College of Physicians of London
ISBN 1 873240 20 1

Typeset by Oxprint Ltd, Aristotle Lane, Oxford OX2 6TR
Printed in Great Britain by Cathedral Press Ltd, Salisbury, Wilts

Membership of the Working Party on Physical Signs of Sexual Abuse in Children

Margaret Turner-Warwick DBE DM PRCP (*President*)

DA Pyke CBE MD FRCP (*Registrar, and Chairman of the Working Party*)

Betty L Priestley FRCP (*Honorary Secretary*) *Consultant Paediatrician, Children's Hospital, Sheffield*

JD Atwell FRCS *Consultant Paediatric and Neonatal Surgeon, Southampton General Hospital*

FN Bamford MD FRCP FFPHM *Reader and Honorary Consultant in Developmental Paediatrics, St Mary's Hospital, Manchester*

PRH Barbor FRCP *Consultant Paediatrician, University Hospital, Nottingham*

C Bate MB *Divisional Police Surgeon to the City of Birmingham*

GD Bell MD FRCP *Consultant Physician and Gastroenterologist, The Ipswich Hospital*

TL Chambers FRCP *Consultant Physician, Paediatric Department, Southmead General Hospital, Bristol*

V Dubowitz MD FRCP *Professor of Paediatrics and Neonatal Medicine, Royal Postgraduate Medical School, Hammersmith Hospital, London*

DK Edmonds FRACOG FRCOG *Consultant Obstetrician and Gynaecologist, Queen Charlotte's and Chelsea Hospital, London*

D Hull FRCP *Professor of Child Health, Medical School, University of Nottingham*

CV Mann FRCS *Formerly Consultant Surgeon for Diseases of the Rectum and Colon, The London Hospital*

Marion V Miles FRCP *Consultant Community Paediatrician, Paddington Community Hospital, London*

Linda J Patterson MRCP (UK) *Consultant Physician, Burnley General Hospital*

Angela J Robinson MRCP (UK) *Consultant Physician in Genito-Urinary Medicine, University College Hospital, London*

Observers
Barbara S Ely MB (to October 1989) (*Department of Health*)
Sonya V Leff MB (*Department of Health*)

In attendance
Linda Connah BA (*Deputy Secretary*)
Elaine M Stephenson BA (*Working Party Secretary*)

Acknowledgements

The Working Party is grateful to the following who gave evidence:

TG Allen-Mersh MD FRCS (*Consultant Surgeon, Westminster Hospital, London*)

GD Clayden MD FRCP (*Consultant Paediatrician, St Thomas's Hospital, London*)

Sir John Dewhurst FRCOG FRCS (Ed) (*Past President, Royal College of Obstetricians and Gynaecologists*)

NAP Evans FRCP (*Consultant Paediatrician, Royal Alexandra Hospital for Sick Children, Brighton*)

Astrid H Heger MD FAAP (*Director, Child Sexual Abuse Program, University of Southern California*)

CJ Hobbs MRCP (UK) (*Consultant Community Paediatrician, St James's University Hospital, Leeds*)

D Jenkins MRCGP (*Past President, Association of Police Surgeons of Great Britain*)

ES Kiff MD FRCS (*Consultant General Surgeon, Withington Hospital, Manchester*)

JON Lawson FRCS (*Consultant Paediatric Surgeon, St Thomas's Hospital, London*)

DM Paul MB (*Past President, British Academy of Forensic Sciences*)

NW Read MD FRCP (*Professor of Gastrointestinal Physiology and Nutrition, University of Sheffield*)

Charlotte M Wright MRCP (UK) (*Northumbria Women's Police Doctors*)

Jane M Wynne MRCP (UK) (*Consultant Community Paediatrician, Leeds General Infirmary, Leeds*)

Contents

Page

Membership of Working Party iii

Acknowledgements iv

1 Introduction 1
Background to the report 1
Membership of the Working Party 1
Terms of reference 1
Limitations of the report 2
Diagnosis of abuse 2

2 Medical evaluation and technique 5
Consent for examination 5
Scope and timing of the examination 7
Genital examination 7
Examination of anus 9
Indications for digital examination of the anal canal
and rectum 10

3 Normal anatomy and variants in appearance
of the female genitalia 11

4 Size of the hymenal orifice and other signs
associated with abuse 15
Size of the hymen 15
Hymenal damage 16
Associated abnormal signs 16
Summary of vulvo-vaginal signs in abuse . . . 17

5 Foreign bodies in the vagina 19

6 Anal abuse 21
Factors affecting physical signs of abuse . . . 21
Variation in incidence of physical findings . . . 21
Perianal erythema and swelling 23

Tyre oedema 23
Anal fissures 23
Venous distension 24
Reflex anal dilatation 25
Anatomy and physiology of the anal canal
and sphincter 25
Buttock separation test 27
Ano-receptive intercourse 28
Prevalence of RAD 28
Constipation and RAD 29
Other conditions associated with anal dilatation . . 30
Mechanism of action of RAD 30
Summary of perianal signs in abuse 31

7 Association of physical with sexual abuse . . 33

8 Healing of physical signs 35

9 Forensic evidence 37
Procedures 37
Chain of evidence 37
Screening for STD 39
DNA techniques 39

10 Sexually transmitted disease in child abuse . . 41
Significance of positive findings 41
Treatment in acute abuse 41

11 Prophylaxis against pregnancy 43

Summary and conclusions 45

References 47

Appendices 49

1 Glossary of terms — anal signs 49
2 An outline approach to medical and forensic investigation
of child sexual abuse 53
3a The significance of forensic medical samples which may
be taken in suspected child sexual abuse . . 55
3b Forensic medical samples: check-list and guidelines . 58
4a Sexually transmitted diseases in child abuse . . 61

Gonorrhoea 61
Chlamydia trachomatis 62
Warts 64
Genital herpes 64
Trichomonas vaginalis 66
Bacterial vaginosis 66
Syphilis 67
HIV infection 67
4b Sexually transmitted disease in child sexual abuse:
Guide to specimen taking and diagnosis . . . 71

1 Introduction

Background to the report

1.1   The Working Party on Physical Signs of Sexual Abuse in Children was set up in December 1988 in response to:

a   The Report of the Inquiry into Child Abuse in Cleveland 1987[1] which recommended that
  — the profession should agree a consistent vocabulary to describe physical signs which may be associated with sexual abuse; 'It is a topic which urgently requires the attention of the medical profession' (p 183).
  — there should be an investigation into the natural history and significance of signs and symptoms which may be associated with child sexual abuse.
  — consideration be given to enquiring into the significance of the phenomenon of anal dilatation.

b   A general concern over major disagreements between branches of the profession regarding the significance of ano-genital signs.

c   The difficulties in legal proceedings caused by the widely divergent views and entrenched positions of some medical experts.

Membership of the Working Party

1.2   Members of the Working Party were invited from all branches of the profession who might reasonably have an interest in the subject. It was agreed, however, that members would make individual contributions rather than act as representatives of defined groups.

1.3   It was known that a Joint Committee of the British Paediatric Association and Association of Police Surgeons was engaged in preparing a glossary of terms and the chairman of that committee, Dr P. Barbor, kindly agreed to join the Working Party to facilitate discussion.

Terms of reference

1.4   The terms of reference of the Working Party were to agree terminology, to describe the range of normal findings, to advise on techniques of examination, to produce evidence of what are the physical signs of child sexual abuse, to assess the significance of these signs **in the light of existing knowledge** and to produce suitable guidelines for the medical and legal professions and others concerned with sexually abused children.

Recommendations for terminology are given in Appendix I.

1.5   The investigation is confined to the ano-genital region plus associated signs.

Limitations of the report

1.6   Most importantly, the Working Party wishes to stress its aware-ness that it is addressing only one aspect of diagnosis—the physical examination. It recognises fully the importance of psychosocial and other aspects including evidence from the child and the carers, behavioural changes, the family background, the presence of risk factors and the general, emotional and developmental status of the child.*

Diagnosis of abuse

1.7   Physical signs of molestation are subtle and rarely diagnostic. Their detection and correct interpretation may be very important in supporting a child's statement or indicating a need for further multi-disciplinary investigation. Many doctors lack such clinical experience and require further training in this aspect of paediatrics.

1.8   **A diagnosis of sexual abuse should rarely, if ever, be made on physical signs alone**. Pregnancy in a child would be an obvious exception to this rule as would the presence of semen on the child, with the possible exception of pubertal boys.

1.9   **A substantial proportion of sexually abused children have no abnormal physical signs. The proportion varies with the types of abuse. Absence of such signs does not imply absence of abuse**.

1.10   Whilst appreciating the importance of recognising abuse when it exists, the Working Party is concerned that too strong an

---

*There is no clear legal definition of 'a child'. For the purposes of this report a child refers to 0–14 years, a young person 14–17 years. In England, Wales and Scotland the age of consent to sexual intercourse is 16 years (Section 14(2) of the Sexual Offences Act 1956, and Section 4(1) of the Sexual Offences (Scotland) Act 1976). Legally therefore, a young person under 16 years cannot give consent.

emphasis may be placed upon physical findings whose precise significance is not yet clear. The genital examination in the following section
applies to girls, since genital abuse in boys usually leaves no signs, or
signs which are easily apparent, eg burn, abrasion, tear of frenulum of
prepuce. Anal signs apply to both sexes.

2 Medical evaluation and technique

2.1   The medical evaluation will include a history taken from the child's carer or social worker, giving information about the child's general health, environment and any behavioural changes. It is important to listen to what the child has to say and it is good practice to record verbatim what both the child and the interviewer say.

2.2   It is very important, as was stressed in the Report of the Inquiry into Child Abuse in Cleveland 1987[1], that a consistent vocabulary is used to describe the appearances of the ano-genital region in order that doctors and others may understand each others' descriptions (see Appendix 1).

2.3   Knowledge of terminology must be linked to skill and experience in recognising what is there to be seen. The difficulties in interpretation of subtle physical findings and the range of normal appearances should not be minimised. The difficulty facing the doctor who is inexperienced in this area is compounded by the often young age of the patient and the brief period of co-operation to be expected during the examination.
The Working Party wishes to stress the importance of encouraging the development of a high level of skill by a small number of doctors in each District. This will require that each of these doctors sees a large number of suspected cases, without which the necessary expertise will not be developed or maintained. The doctors involved should be accustomed to communicating well with children and may be paediatricians in hospitals or in the community, police surgeons, or other doctors with a special interest and skill. They will need to keep meticulous records, provide forensic samples where indicated, attend case conferences, present reports, and give evidence in courts.

Consent for examination

2.4   Where there is concern that sexual abuse has taken place, **consent for examination** should be obtained from the parent(s) and from the child when age and understanding make this appropriate.
When a child is brought to be seen by a doctor it is normally expected that the doctor will examine as much of the child as is felt necessary (implied consent). Failure to do so may be regarded as negligent. It is the custom of paediatricians to carry out a full examination of the child,

and a request such as 'May I have a look at her now?' almost always receives a positive response.

Examination of the ano-genital region will be appropriate when a child presents following an allegation of abuse, or when the presenting complaints are such as may be positively associated with abuse, or when the nature of the complaint involves the ano-genital region, eg localised pain, irritation, discharge, urinary tract infection, constipation, blood loss.

The question of obtaining informed consent may present difficulties if the doctor wishes to take specimens for forensic examination. This would normally follow an allegation of abuse within the preceding 72 hours.

In the case of a child who is a Ward of Court, the permission of a High Court Judge is required. The situation will change when the new Children Act comes into force in 1991 and wardship proceedings are likely to become less common.*

---

*Child Protection

1. The law relating to the protection of children is strengthened in Part V of the Children Act, which comes into force in October 1991. The aim is to protect children from harm, including sexual abuse and forms of ill treatment which are not physical, yet avoid the child suffering harm caused by unwarranted intervention in family life. Whilst the interests of the child are paramount, and the courts are given wide powers to intervene, a new principle is that orders should not be made unless failure to do so would be to the detriment of the child.

2. To issue an *emergency protection order*, the court must be satisfied that, unprotected, the child is likely to suffer significant ill treatment or impairment of health or development. The order lasts for eight days and may be extended once only, for a further seven days; and there is provision for parents to challenge the order. The order may be made whilst the Local Authority is carrying out an investigation, or when an investigation is frustrated by the officer being denied access to the child, or where access is required as a matter of urgency. The applicant is given parental responsibility, and unless the court directs otherwise, must allow reasonable contact with the parents while the order is in force.

3. *Child assessment orders* are issued where there is concern about the child's welfare and the parents are proving uncooperative, yet there is no case for an emergency protection order. The assessment order may last up to seven days only and is intended to assist the local authority carry out its investigative duty. This order does not involve removing the child from the parental home, but enables the applicant to achieve medical, psychiatric or other assessment of the child.

Scope and timing of the examination

2.5   Physical examination should include measurements of height and weight, and assessment of behaviour and development. Examination of the genitalia should always be done as part of a general examination, and usually at the end.

2.6   Associated signs of abuse should be looked for, including injuries within the mouth, 'love bites', teeth marks and bruising.

2.7   The particular pattern of grip marks suggesting restraint for sexual abuse should be looked for (para 7.2).

2.8   The examination should be carried out without delay when the abuse is thought to have occurred within the previous 72 hours. In the case of a young child, considerable reassurance will be needed and when the abuse has not been recent, the examination may be delayed, for example, until the following day. In order to avoid further emotional distress to the child, no force or restraint should be used.

2.9   Very young children are often best examined on their mothers' laps. It should be appreciated that the shape of the hymen will appear different when a girl is examined sitting on her mother's lap and when she is examined supine.

Genital examination

2.10   The recommended position for the genital examination[2] of most girls is supine in the 'frog-legged' position, with the hips flexed and the soles of the feet touching (Figure 1). For children under 3 years old, the mother may hold the child in this position on her lap.

2.11   The prone knee-chest position is not generally recommended because there is very limited experience in this country in interpreting the appearances so produced. However, if there is a problem in visualising the posterior margin of the hymen adequately, eg with the fimbriated variety, this may be more easily accomplished in the prone posture because it allows relaxation of the pelvic floor muscles which tends to give apparent increase in the antero-posterior diameter of the hymen.

2.12   Digital examination of the vagina is not indicated in young children unless there is specific reason, for example:

 i Bleeding or other indication of possible vaginal wall injury, in which case it is probably preferable to examine the vagina using a small cystoscope under general anaesthetic.

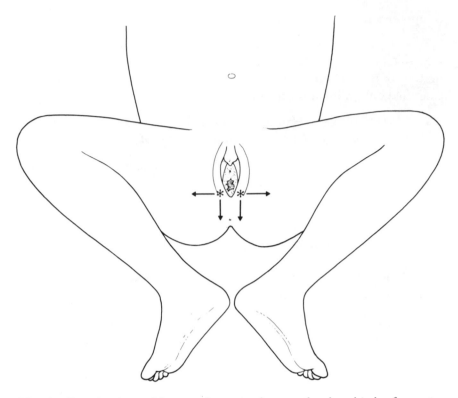

Fig. 1. *Examination position: gentle traction between thumb and index finger at posterior edge of labia majora to show irregular torn hymen.*

    ii A story of repeated penile penetration, where it may be important to assess the capacity and length of the vagina and the smoothness of its walls. This would apply mainly to post-pubertal children or young persons.

    iii Some experienced clinicians have found gentle insertion of a small finger helpful in the older child, in assessing elasticity of the hymen.

2.13   The external genitalia should be examined carefully in a good light. The use of an otoscope lens with the speculum removed gives a ×5 magnification. The labia majora, labia minora, urethra, perihymenal regions, posterior fourchette, vestibule, hymen and what is visible of the vagina should be inspected for signs of recent or old injuries. The vaginal walls are *not* specifically examined unless there is a likelihood of injury.

2.14   In order to visualise the hymen, the techniques of labial separation or labial traction may be used. These give very different hymenal orifice dimensions. When the labia are simply separated, the hymenal tissue will often appear closed or in close apposition. A gaping orifice is suggestive of abuse. In order to assess the configuration of the hymenal orifice, it is usually necessary to exert gentle labial traction, ie the posterior ends of the labia majora are grasped gently between thumb and forefinger and pulled gently towards the child's feet and slightly backwards. This usually allows a clear demonstration of the urethra, the periurethral support ligaments and the hymen.

2.15   Glass rods[3] have been used by some physicians to assess the hymenal size. This is not generally recommended since the tissue is dynamic and elastic, rendering measurement in this way unreliable. The glass rods, or bulbs, are however very useful in enabling the edge of the hymen to be examined. This method may reveal a previously undetected split in the hymen.

2.16   A colposcope adapted for examination of the external genitalia, with an in-built measuring device and camera, is used in some centres. It gives an accurate measure of the hymenal orifice and can be very helpful in allowing the vascular pattern to be demonstrated. The normal symmetrical lace-like pattern can then easily be distinguished from the irregular 'smudged' vascularity when abuse has occurred. Care is needed in the interpretation of colposcopic findings. It has been reported[4] to show up minor genital trauma not otherwise detected in a small proportion of girls referred for assessment of abuse, but there is uncertainty about the incidence of minor findings in a normal population. A colposcope is not at present recommended for general use.

Examination of anus

2.17   Examination of the anus includes the following steps:

  i The anal and perianal areas are examined with the child lying in the left lateral position, curled up with hips and knees flexed, the head resting on a pillow.

  ii The buttocks are gently separated using both hands. This action alone is likely to apply some traction to the anus. The examiner then pauses for 30 seconds, to see whether the anal canal opens. This has been described as the 'buttock separation' or 'lateral buttock traction test', and the opening of the anal canal as 'reflex anal dilatation' (RAD) (paras 6.34–6.40).

iii The perianal region is inspected for signs of inflammation, injury or venous congestion.

iv Gentle palpation of, and traction on, the anal verge allows some assessment of tone of the external sphincter and inspection for fissures.

v The fineness and symmetry of the anal verge radiating skin folds are also noted.

vi A digital examination of the anus is not usually necessary but may be performed to allow assessment of tone, elasticity and contractility of the sphincter, especially if chronic abuse is suspected. It may also disclose the presence of a stool beyond the rectal ampulla. (See paras 2.18–2.20.)

Indications for digital examination of the anal canal and rectum

2.18   This is another contentious subject. The majority of paediatricians take the view that fingers should not be inserted into any orifice unless there is a clear idea of the usefulness of the extra information to be gained thereby, since the procedure itself is unpleasant. Some reserve a digital examination for the occurrence of RAD and uncertainty about the presence of stool in the rectum. An attempt is made to assess the anal tone by palpation and gentle traction on the anal verge, without a digital examination of the anal canal.

2.19   Forensic physicians/police surgeons feel there is a need to carry out a rectal examination in order to assess anal tone, and in particular the elasticity and reduced contractility likely to accompany chronic anal abuse.

2.20   Each doctor will have an individual opinion as to the help to be gained by digital examination and will act accordingly. However, situations in which it may prove helpful are:

a to ensure there is no other cause for physical signs, eg rectal polyp causing bleeding or discharge;

b to assess anal tone when this is suspected to be abnormal;

c for further information as to the presence in the rectum of a stool which may have been hidden out of view during inspection through a dilated anus.

3 Normal anatomy and variants in appearance of the female genitalia

3.1   There is considerable variation in appearance according to the age of the child. The newborn often shows the effect of passive oestrogenic stimulation, ie swollen and oedematous hymen, copious white vaginal secretions, reddened labia minora and sometimes a hymenal tag. In the neonate the labia majora lie laterally, exposing the labia minora. During early infancy the labia majora become plump and gradually fold across the introitus to form a protective pad of fat.

3.2   Congenital absence of the hymen is sometimes considered in differential diagnosis. However, experts in the field have been unable to recall ever seeing a case, and Jenny et al.[5] report on the examination of 1,131 infant girls, when 1,131 hymens were identified. Of the infants examined, 3–4% had normal anatomic variants, such as tags and transverse hymenal bands. In the absence of major genito-urinary abnormality, hymenal tissue should be present in prepubescent girls.

3.3   The hymenal configuration is commonly annular. Variants include a posterior rim hymen which is deficient anteriorly and a fimbriated hymen with redundant edges shaped like a tulip, a characteristic seen more often in very young girls (Figs 2 and 3). There is variation in different authors' experience as to whether the annular hymen or the posterior rim hymen is the most common type. The American literature indicates that the posterior rim hymen is the most frequently found, for example, 75–80% of the girls seen at a large referral centre for vulvovaginal complaints and abuse had the posterior rim variant. A second group of 124 prepubertal girls[6] referred for gynaecological examination over a two-year period showed the posterior rim variant in 45%, annular in 27%, and fimbriated in 20%. This does not necessarily represent the distribution in a normal population. The author wondered whether gradual coercive dilatation might convert an annular or fimbriated hymen into a posterior rim, since this variant is commoner in older girls.

3.4   Variations of the normal include:

a A bifid hymen, with a narrow strip of tissue dividing the orifice into two, often unequal, parts. The vagina may also be septate and associated with a bicornuate uterus.

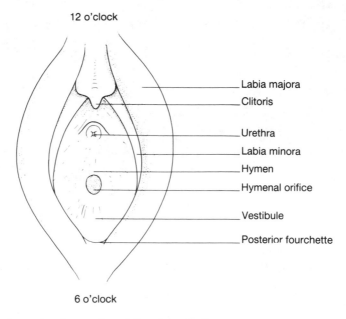

Fig. 2. *Anatomy of pre-pubertal female genitalia.*

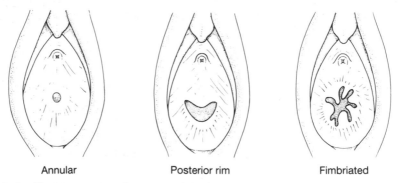

Fig. 3. *Variations in configuration of the hymen.*

b A microperforate or imperforate hymen.

c A hymenal cyst.

d Fusion of the labia minora. The precise aetiology is unclear. The condition may be acquired within a few months of birth and is unlikely once the girl is secreting oestrogen. It is not uncommon in young infants but becomes infrequent in older girls.[7] An association with frictional trauma has been suggested, as in abuse or vigorous masturbation, but is unproven.

e An enlarged clitoris is described as possibly resulting from masturbation but this too is doubtful. It is also seen in association with ambiguous genitalia, which may be a manifestation of masculinisation of a female fetus, eg congenital adrenal hyperplasia, incomplete masculinisation of a male fetus, or true hermaphroditism.

f Appearances of the genitalia are usually normal in girls with chromosomal abnormalities, unless Y material is present.

g The anus may be anteriorly displaced and associated with a short perineum, predisposing to fissure.

3.5   Variations of normal appearance that may lead to confusion with sexual abuse include the common finding of a posterior rim hymen deficient anteriorly, and a midline translucent channel running between the fourchette and the anal margin; this is associated with the backward migration of the anus during early development and sometimes referred to as a 'congenital fissure'. There may be a midline area of pallor, presumably avascular, which may be confused with scarring.

3.6   Lichen sclerosus et atrophicus is a condition which has been confused with sexual abuse.[8] Because of the increasing interest in ano-genital complaints, it is being recognised more frequently in young girls. The epidermis shows pale patches, starting as pink to ivory flat-topped papules which coalesce into pearly plaques with wrinkling and increased fragility. It may contain vascular or purpuric areas and ecchymoses. Fissures are common in association with increased fragility and susceptibility to vulvo-vaginitis. Usual symptoms include pruritus, discharge, soreness and bleeding. There may be genetic, hormonal and auto-immune factors involved. The possibility of frictional trauma from sexual abuse[9] being an aetiological factor in some cases has, as yet, no evidence to support it.

3.7   The changes in ano-genital lichen sclerosus et atrophicus are restricted in area, rarely extending laterally beyond the margins of the labia majora but commonly extending to surround the anus in a characteristic figure of eight distribution. If there is any bruising outside these limits another explanation should be sought. Further, although the condition responds variably to fluorinated steroids, it is unlikely that all signs of it will clear within a short period of time, whereas it is commonly the case that when sexual abuse ceases the associated physical signs heal quite quickly.

3.8   The appearance of the hymen changes with age. At one year of age it is often sleeve-like, fleshy and redundant. At around 3 years of age there may be a longitudinal fold anteriorly, with flaps of redundant hymen at 11 and 1 o'clock, overlapping each other. With increasing age the hymenal membrane becomes thinner. As puberty approaches the hymen assumes a sleeve-like or flower-like appearance (fimbriated variety).

3.9   Waxy localised thickenings or 'bumps' may occur inferiorly at the edge of the hymen, possibly representing lymphoid aggregates, as a variant of normal. The appearance contrasts with that of a bump caused by trauma, in which case the hymen would appear disrupted. Bumps associated with abuse are also found in the posterior margin.[10]

3.10   A cleft or notch at 12 o'clock is a normal variant, as is a notch at 11 o'clock and 1 o'clock with a crescentic hymen (posterior rim). A notch may also be a result of trauma but in this case is likely to be associated with scarring of the hymen.

3.11   Vaginal septal remnants may remain as a projection or smooth non-scarred bump on the hymen.

3.12   Hymenal elasticity increases with pubertal development. It appears that the hymenal orifice may be so elastic in some girls that the orifice may remain deceptively small despite penetration having occurred.

4 Size of the hymenal orifice and other signs associated with abuse

Size of the hymen

4.1   Clearly the relative sizes of the object inserted and the recipient will be important. It is likely that penile penetration in a five-year-old girl, for example, will result in significant damage to the hymen, the posterior fourchette and possibly the perineum. However in a recent report[11] of 18 sexually abused girls, where the perpetrator admitted to vaginal penetration, the genitalia appeared normal or showed only non-specific changes in four. These girls were aged 5, 6, 7 and 11 years and the interval between the abusive episode and the examination was less than one week in three cases. It therefore seems that, rarely, findings may be absent even in young girls, where both victim and assailant describe penetration.

4.2   The size of the hymenal orifice has been the subject of a great deal of discussion and disagreement, the most commonly held view being that an orifice greater than 4 mm in the pre-pubertal child is strongly correlated with abuse.[12,13] This measurement is of the apparent hymenal size when the labia are separated without traction. Labial traction will however enlarge the horizontal diameter of the hymenal orifice.

4.3   It is likely that there is some increase in diameter with increasing age, and one suggestion by Woodling[14] is that from infancy to 4 years the maximum diameter is 4 mm. After 5 years of age the maximum diameter in millimetres is roughly equal to the child's age. In this study the diameter was measured transversely, between 3 and 9 o'clock in the supine position.

4.4   Some experienced observers hold the view that a skilled examiner may achieve a wider hymenal diameter, since he or she is more likely to achieve relaxation in the child. This makes it difficult to be dogmatic over hymenal size, which may also vary with position and technique. Nevertheless, an individual examiner may find hymenal measurement a helpful guide within his/her own service.

4.5   At puberty, the horizontal hymenal diameter is approximately 1 cm. **It is generally agreed that an orifice of greater than 1 cm is not**

seen in normal pre-pubertal children, and that a hymenal size of 1.5 cm in association with other evidence of trauma would be highly suggestive of abuse. **It cannot, however, be used as the sole basis for a diagnosis of abuse but may be supportive**.

Hymenal damage

4.6   An attenuated scarred hymen is a sign of damage due to the hymenal tissue being rubbed or worn away by chronic abuse. This appearance is never seen in normal children.

4.7   Transections or lacerations of the hymen may be circumferential but are commonly at 5–7 o'clock[2,10] and often involve the posterior fourchette. They are associated with penile penetration. When this has been repeated, synechiae or bridging scars may develop. A laceration may extend from the hymen to involve the posterior vaginal wall.

4.8   Digital penetration of the hymen is more likely to cause abrasions or tears between 3 and 9 o'clock anteriorly. Similarly, accidental trauma is likely to affect the ventral area or periurethral area, with lateral bruising and usually without penetration of the hymen.[10]

4.9   In a study of 205 pre-pubertal girls who had been sexually abused,[15] of those girls who reported penile penetration, 86% showed definite signs of abuse (tears, or presence of sperm) (49 of 57 girls), whereas of those who reported digital abuse, 16% only showed definite signs (12 of 74 girls). The genitalia appeared normal in 3.5% of girls reporting penile contact and in 57% of those complaining of digital assault.

Associated abnormal signs

4.10   Abnormalities of the genital region in association with abuse may be minor non-specific findings of the sort which may also occur in non-abused children as a result of inflammation, infection and poor hygiene. These changes include erythema, vascular congestion of the labia and vestibule, marked friability of the perineal skin with easy fissuring, vaginal discharge and fusion of the labia minora.

4.11   In a small child, compression of the soft tissues by the penis against the body margins of the pelvic outlet produces bruising of the labia with associated abrasion and swelling.[16]

4.12   **It must be remembered that there may be no physical findings in as many as two-thirds of the children seen for suspected sexual abuse.**

4.13   Pregnancy in a child or young person under 16 years of age indicates either abuse or unlawful sexual intercourse.

Summary of vulvo-vaginal signs in abuse

4.14   Vulvo-vaginal signs may be summarised as follows:

1. **Diagnostic** of blunt force penetrating trauma.

a   Laceration or scars in the hymen, which may extend to the posterior vaginal wall.

b   Attenuation of the hymen with loss of hymenal tissue.

2. **Supportive**, but not diagnostic.

a   Enlarged hymenal opening (paras 4.1–4.5).

b   Notch in the hymenal edge which may be associated with scarring. A notch may be normal at 11 and 1 o'clock in a crescentic hymen, without scarring (para 3.10).

c   A bump on the hymen, plus some disruption. Care is needed to differentiate from an innocent bump or tag (para 3.9).

d   Localised erythema and oedema, pouting urethra and hymen; minor abrasions suggestive of vulval coitus.[14]

e   Posterior fourchette. A mounded scar is abnormal and may follow a splitting or shearing injury. Labial fusion may be associated with any irritation/infection in the area such as may occur in vulval coitus or more innocently with napkin rash.

5 Foreign bodies in the vagina

5.1   Foreign bodies in the vagina are unusual in children[16] and will result in bleeding as a predominant symptom,[17] followed next in frequency by offensive discharge.

5.2   They may be inserted innocently by the child—often little macerated pieces of toilet tissue—but, especially if recurrent, deserve consideration as to the possibility of previous sexual abuse.

5.3   Use of tampons by post-pubertal girls is not associated with bruising, abrasion, laceration or other hymenal damage.[18] Repeated use may lead to minor stretching of the orifice.

5.4   The majority of pre-pubertal girls presenting with vaginal discharge do not have a foreign body, or any disease or any sinister explanation for the symptom. In these cases, assessment and reassurance is all that is required.

6 Anal abuse

Factors affecting physical signs of abuse

6.1   Child sexual abuse may involve the anal region in a variety of acts including touching, rubbing, sucking, licking, kissing and penetration of the anus by tongue, finger, penis or any suitably shaped object. Clearly, some forms of contact will leave no physical signs and others will depend upon the position of the child relative to the abuser, and the size of the object inserted relative to the size of the orifice.

6.2   Other factors influencing physical findings include the degree of force used, the use of lubricant, the frequency of abuse and the period of time which has elapsed since the last episode of abuse.

6.3   Many of the physical signs are minor ones, which can be used to corroborate a child's story of abuse but which are not, by themselves, indicative of abuse. When found in association with other grounds for suspicion, they may be sufficient to justify a **multi-disciplinary investigation.*** This is regarded as essential to the management of a case of suspected child abuse.

Variation in incidence of physical findings

6.4   The incidence of these signs varies in different series and there appears to be a considerable variability of medical findings in children examined for sexual abuse in different parts of the world. It has been suggested that this may reflect the much greater awareness of abuse in the USA which should bring children to the physician early in the history of the abuse 'before many physical findings exist'.[20] Also, different techniques of examination have been used.

6.5   Another factor which will influence the incidence of physical findings is the existence of 'open access' clinics and the practice of bringing children very early for medical examination, rather than

---

*No single profession or agency should take full responsibility for the assessment and diagnosis of child sexual abuse. It is strongly recommended[19] that full inter-agency co-operation should take place, involving health, social services, police and, where appropriate, voluntary organisations. Social services have a statutory duty to protect children and young persons.

delaying until a psychosocial investigation has been completed, when some of the transient signs will have disappeared.

6.6   In order to illustrate some of this variability and areas of overlap between abused and presumed non-abused children, two papers are discussed here in detail. In a series of 337 probable or confirmed cases reported from Leeds,[21] 143 (42%) had positive anal findings. The percentage frequencies of individual signs in the group with anal findings are shown below:

Perianal erythema	53%
Fissures or tears	53%
Reflex anal dilatation	42%
Laxity	38%
Venous congestion	24%
Swelling ('tyre')	8%
Scars, tags	8%
Genital warts	4%

Anal twitching, funnelling, haematoma and bruising were also observed.

6.7   In contrast, a recent American series from Fresno, California[22] provides data from 267 children judged unlikely to have been abused. The following findings were reported in this supposedly normal population.

Perianal erythema	41%	
Fissures	0%	
Reflex anal dilatation	49%	*(15% of the total by 30 secs 26% of the total by 2 mins)*
Venous congestion	52%	*(after 2 mins observation)*
Increased pigmentation	30%	
Wedge shaped smooth areas in the midline	26%	
Tags or folds (anterior)	11%	
Warts	0%	

6.8   Although this reported incidence in a group of presumed non-abused children is somewhat surprising, the two series differ in a number of fundamental respects. The Leeds children were examined in the lateral position or, if very young, on their mothers' laps. The period of observation was around 30 secs. The Fresno children were examined in the prone knee–chest position and the periods of observation varied from 15 secs to 8 minutes, with a mean of 4 minutes. Thus, whilst venous congestion was present in 7% of the children at the onset, this had increased to 73% after 4 minutes in the knee–chest position. A prolonged inspection is likely to cause distress and **the Working Party strongly recommends that the period of peri-anal inspection as described should not normally exceed 30 seconds** (para 2.17–2.20).

6.9   Significant abnormal findings in the Fresno series were scars, skin tags outside the midline, an irregular dilated anal orifice, a prominent anal verge and reflex anal dilatation greater than 20 mm.

6.10   It may be significant that in this group of children the possibility of abuse was discounted by a structured interview with the parents. The children were not themselves interviewed. Yet in a study of children attending a psychological clinic, it was found that the proportion of children disclosing abuse increased markedly with directed questioning, ie from 7% to 31%.[23] It is therefore possible that some abused children may have inadvertently been included in the 'normal' sample.

In addition, the conduct and timing of the medical examinations differed so markedly in the two studies as to make comparisons invalid.

Perianal erythema and swelling

6.11   Perianal erythema varies in extent according to the degree of friction involved. Thus, in intracrural intercourse, the erythema extends forwards to involve the perineum, labia and upper inner aspects of the thighs. Reddening of the perianal region may also occur in association with poor hygiene, faecal soiling or seepage, irritation from thread worms, napkin eruption and skin disorders, eg moniliasis, lichen sclerosus et atrophicus.

Tyre oedema

6.12   Perianal swelling, resembling a 'tyre' of oedema, is thought to represent post-traumatic oedema and as such is likely to be found for a very brief period, eg 24–36 hours after the injury or traumatic event.

Anal fissures

6.13   Anal fissures or tears represent breaks in the perianal skin or mucosa, often extending from the skin up into the anal canal and anal mucosa. The fissure is usually triangular in shape, with the apex within the anal canal. The edges of the lower part of the fissure are pulled apart by the corrugator cutis ani muscle. Fissures resulting from constipation cannot be distinguished by appearance from those due to abuse. The appearance of a fissure does not give information as to its cause.

Fissures may be acute or chronic with rolled edges, single or multiple and superficial or deep. Fissures are painful in the acute situation and may result in anal spasm and very painful defaecation. However this is often not the case with chronic fissures resulting from abuse. Deep fissures are likely to heal with scarring, possibly with a skin tag representing overgrowth of the skin in the healing process.

6.14   There are differing opinions as to the significance of anal fissures in relation to abuse and it is likely that the age range of the subjects examined is important here. Thus, McCann[22] in his study of 267 presumed normal children — mainly older than infancy, with average age of 5 years 7 months — found no fissures. Hobbs and Wynne[21] state that fissures are unusual, that even in a constipated child a single fissure is exceptional, that scars are rare and that more than two fissures have — in their experience — followed only abuse. This does not include tiny superficial cracks at the anal verge, possibly resulting from scratching due to threadworm, napkin rash or diarrhoea.

6.15   In contrast, in a study in Brighton of 136 children with mild to moderate constipation, Evans *et al.*[24] reported that 35 children (25.7%) had anal fissures, mostly anteriorly placed. Nineteen children had multiple fissures, ie 10 had two fissures, at least one of which was outside the midline in each child and eight had multiple fissures, including two children who had fissures all round the anus.

It is also important to note that in children with constipation, an underlying cause may be anal stenosis with an anteriorly placed anus. This may result in severe anterior tears which may be refractory to healing.

6.16   In our opinion, **acute anal fissures are not unusual in children who have not been abused.** They may be associated with constipation, threadworms, napkin rash, diarrhoea, eczema and lichen sclerosus et atrophicus. They are usually midline in either the anterior or posterior position.

Venous distension

6.17   Venous distension of the vascular plexus underlying the perianal skin produces a dark purple-blue discoloration which may be crescentic or may surround the anus. It is suggested that any persisting congestion is abnormal, though not necessarily associated with abuse. Dilated veins around the anus are—in the experience of some coloproctologists and paediatric surgeons—not abnormal, although their persistence probably is.

6.18   Veins may distend in association with defaecation, but then would be expected to subside.

Engorged veins are common in small babies with constipation and after defaecation.

Piles (internal haemorrhoids) are very unusual in childhood and when they do occur there is a strong family history. They appear at 3, 7 and 11 o'clock and are so infrequent that fewer than one case per annum would be seen by a paediatric surgeon.

6.19   In sexual abuse, venous congestion may extend beyond the perianal area and may be one of the last signs to resolve.

6.20   It is noted in paediatric surgical practice that an anal stretch procedure under general anaesthetic—eg to admit two fingers in a 2-year-old child—does not usually result in significant venous distension in the perianal area and the anal size usually contracts back to normal within a few days. It is not, as far as is known, followed by reflex anal dilatation but this response may not have been sought.

Reflex anal dilatation

6.21   Reflex anal dilatation (RAD) is an incompletely understood phenomenon which needs to be interpreted with caution and in context.

Anatomy and physiology of the anal canal and sphincter

6.22   The anal canal is that part of the terminal large bowel surrounded by the internal anal sphincter. The rectum extends from the upper margin of the anal canal to the recto-sigmoid junction. The anal canal is 1.8 cm long at birth, 2.5 cm long at 2 years and 3 cm in the adult. The rectum increases from 7 cm at birth to 11.5 cm at 2 years and 14 cm in the adult. There is therefore relatively little increase in length after 2 years of age.

6.23   The pelvic diaphragm consists of voluntary muscle. As the rectum, with its involuntary smooth muscle, passes through the pelvic floor it is surrounded by a sleeve of voluntary muscle which forms the external anal sphincter. This is supplied by the pudendal nerve below the pelvic floor.

The lower part of the circular muscle of the terminal large bowel is expanded to form the internal anal sphincter, which is under involuntary control. It is supplied by the parasympathetic and sympathetic nerves and by the myenteric plexus.

6.24   Closure of the anal canal at rest is the result of the internal sphincter action plus the close apposition of the six major folds of mucosa and submucosal muscle in the anal canal.

6.25   The ano-rectal reflexes include:

i The cutaneo-anal reflex, in which the external sphincter contracts in response to perineal touch.

ii The recto-anal reflex in which distension of the rectum induces relaxation of the internal anal sphincter. This is mediated through the myenteric plexus but heavily modulated by activity in the sympathetic nerves. Rectal distension may also induce rectal contractions and contraction of the external sphincter, both via a spinal reflex.

iii The ano-rectal reflex, whereby stimulation or distension of the anal canal induces a propagating contraction of the rectum, which may in turn relax the internal anal sphincter. This reflex is present in paraplegic patients with a high spinal injury and also in infants. It is difficult to demonstrate in adults and may disappear during infancy.

6.26   When a rectal wave of contraction results in a descending column of faeces and relaxation of the internal sphincter, the external sphincter may contract and the urge to defaecate then passes until a convenient time.

6.27   Weakness of the external anal sphincter may therefore lead to urgency of defaecation, since contraction in the external sphincter is the usual short-term defence mechanism maintaining continence. When external sphincter function is impaired, traction on the anal verge will stretch the internal sphincter ring and cause it to give way so that the anus opens widely.

6.28   Weakness of the internal sphincter may result in leakage of flatus or mucus, with faecal staining and possibly pruritus ani. There may be urgency and whether this results in incontinence will depend upon the strength of contraction of the external sphincter.

6.29   Weakness of both sphincters results in faecal incontinence.

6.30   Distension of the anal canal inhibits tonic contraction of the internal sphincter. Contraction of the external sphincter is transiently increased but during defaecation these contractile responses to distension of the rectum and anus are inhibited centrally, leading to unrestricted evacuation of the rectum once the process has commenced.

6.31   The effect of anal stretching in producing relaxation of the internal sphincter has been clearly demonstrated in patients with paraplegia.[25] In paraplegics the reflexes can be examined without alteration by cortical influence.

6.32   Anal distension has been shown to be a powerful stimulus to internal sphincter relaxation and a similar effect is produced by traction on the ano-rectal ring. Digital stimulation of the rectum has in the past been practised in paraplegics in order to facilitate evacuation of the bowel. The external sphincter is inhibited and the whole sphincter mass can be felt to give way after an initial contraction.

6.33   Attempts to penetrate the anus lead to contraction of the voluntary external sphincter, but this muscle is heavily influenced by higher nervous control so that excitatory or inhibitory responses to stimuli may be learnt, eg the muscle may be relaxed during ano-receptive intercourse, which would otherwise be painful and very difficult.

Buttock separation test

6.34   The buttock separation test, in the left lateral position, involves gentle parting of the buttocks to display the anal area. Observation is continued for 30 secs, during which time the external sphincter contracts briefly and is often subsequently seen to relax. It is commonly believed that the external sphincter is unable to maintain contraction for longer than 30 secs but in adults there is some evidence that contraction can be maintained up to 3 minutes. A positive test involves a dynamic relaxation of the internal sphincter as well as the external so that the anus presents a cylindrical hole with a clear view into the rectum, ie reflex anal dilatation. The scientific basis for describing this reaction as a reflex is lacking. The term has been retained in this report because it is frequently used in clinical practice and to avoid ambiguity.

6.35   Theoretically, when the external sphincter has relaxed, buttock traction might then be exerted on the internal sphincter ring, which might then relax in turn. It has been suggested that it might be possible to pull apart the internal sphincter using digital traction on the perianal skin. This is unlikely, using an acceptable degree of pressure in older children. In younger children with a short anal canal it may be possible, although unusual, to open up the anal canal with sustained pressure. When sphincter tone is impaired, as in neurogenic conditions such as spina bifida and sacral agenesis, opening of the internal sphincter may be more easily achieved.

6.36   Reflex anal dilatation is a sign which has been recognised for some years by forensic physicians. It is elicited during the lateral buttock traction test or buttock separation test and has been referred to as the 'O' sign,[25] which it was thought may sometimes be seen in passive homosexuals.

Ano-receptive intercourse

6.37   A study was carried out on adults indulging in ano-receptive intercourse in order to investigate the statement that anal sphincter tone is reduced after repeated anal abuse.[16] Sixteen men who had regular ano-receptive intercourse were compared with 17 heterosexual age matched controls. Of the homosexuals, 56% admitted to minor symptoms, mainly a sense of urgency. This appeared to be age related, suggesting the pelvic floor muscles may become laxer with age and/or number of episodes of penetration. There was a slight reduction in resting anal pressure in the homosexuals (internal sphincter activity) and this effect appeared to be dose related in terms of promiscuity, possibly due to temporary stretching of the fibres. However, the maximum squeeze pressure (external sphincter) was unchanged. Unfortunately, it was not possible to relate the findings to the time interval between the most recent episode of intercourse and the examination. Reflex anal dilatation was not seen in any of these adults.

Prevalence of RAD

6.38   Hobbs and Wynne[21,28] reported RAD to be present in 42% of anally abused children and claim that it is an important abnormal finding in the context of abuse. Reflex anal dilatation has been reported in various frequencies as follows:

i Hobbs and Wynne[21,28]	4% of 1368 children referred for suspicion of all kinds of abuse and neglect.	
	18% of 337 children with probable or certain sexual abuse.	
	42% of sexually abused children with anal signs.	
ii Northumbria policewomen, Ellis-Fraser and Wright[29]	8.5% of 224 children referred for investigation of possible sexual abuse.	

iii	McCann *et al.*[22]	49% of 267 normal controls (mean dia 10 mm) (15% during the first 30 secs)
iv	Stanton and Sunderland[30]	14% of 200 presumed non-abused children attending – a community health clinic (78) – a general paediatric clinic (101) – a renal clinic (21) (5 mm to 35 mm diameter)
v	Priestley[31]	4% of 100 children seen in general paediatric practice with no suggestion of abuse.
vi	Evans *et al.*[24]	18% of 136 children with mild to moderate constipation showed full or partial dilatation (full in 8%)
vii	Clayden[32]	15% of 129 children with severe chronic constipation had 'visibly relaxed sphincters' (and had received enemas, suppositories)

Constipation and RAD

6.39   Hobbs and Wynne conclude that RAD greater than 0.5 cm (without the simultaneous passage of flatus) does not occur in normal children examined in the left lateral position and observed for 30 secs. McCann *et al.* found RAD in 49% of their supposedly normal population examined for up to 8 minutes in the knee–chest position. The observation period was prolonged and, in the view of the Working Party, unacceptably so, but 30% of those who dilated did so within the first 30 secs, ie 15% of the total.

   Whilst it is clear that the knee–chest position produces a different appearance in some children from the more usual left lateral position, McCann's 15% within 30 seconds is very similar to Stanton's 14%, Clayden's 15% and Evans' 8–18%.

6.40   There is some evidence from the studies of McCann *et al.*, Stanton *et al.*, Evans and Clayden that RAD is commoner when stool is present in the rectum. This may not necessarily be visible by simply looking through the dilated sphincter.

6.41   The association of constipation in children and reflex anal dilatation merits consideration. A full and chronically distended rectum is likely to lead to internal sphincter relaxation with soiling. Chronic straining at stool may also lead to some weakness of the anal sphincter. 'A visibly relaxed anus' has been described[32] in 20 of 129 children with severe constipation. These children had also received treatment by enema or suppository which may have modified their response, but it was felt that this reflected the greater degree of faecal loading in the group with relaxed sphincters as compared with the rest of the children studied. Although no child was seen with a dilated sphincter without faecal loading, anal dilatation was not routinely sought by the buttock separation test as described. Therefore some children with a dynamic reflex dilatation response to buttock separation may have been missed. Evans found full RAD in 11 out of 136 mildly constipated children. Six out of these 11 showed faecal loading. It appears that children with faecal loading may or may not show RAD, and RAD may or may not be related to the degree of loading.

Reflex anal dilatation is rarely seen by doctors treating adult patients for constipation, incontinence or more unusual ano-rectal conditions.

Other conditions associated with anal dilatation

6.42   Reflex anal dilatation may sometimes be found in children with Crohn's disease. There are a number of other situations in which anal dilatation, though not the dynamic response, may be seen in children. These include general anaesthesia, especially in infants and toddlers, who have not yet developed continence. It is possible that the response may be different at different developmental stages, ie the neonate, the toddler without bowel control, the older child and the adult.

Neurogenic bowel problems with a weak external sphincter may result in anal laxity, as may recurrent rectal prolapse. Anal dilatation may also be seen in seriously ill children (eg on a ventilator; in intensive care; in haemolytic uraemic syndrome) and is a frequent finding post-mortem when the sphincters are relaxed.

6.43   **It is particularly important that appearances under these conditions, which are already distressing, are not misinterpreted as pointers to abuse.**[33]

Mechanism of action of RAD

6.44   It has been suggested, in evidence presented to the Working Party, that some children are able to relax the external sphincter, or have a weak external sphincter (eg rarely in spina bifida occulta or in neuro-muscular disease). In these, the buttock separation test may then exert traction on the ano-rectal ring, leading to relaxation of the internal sphincter and RAD. Read holds the view that anything which causes weakness of the external sphincter may give rise to RAD. If the internal sphincter is damaged in addition then the anal canal may be already open and there will be no dynamic reflex dilatation. If the internal sphincter alone is impaired — an unusual occurrence — and the external sphincter intact, reflex dilatation will not occur.

A more widely held belief is that it is damage to the *internal* sphincter which is likely to result in RAD. This controversy is at present insoluble since, for ethical and practical reasons, the relevant studies in children have not been done.

6.45   **The Working Party stresses that a lax, possibly dilated anus is different from an anus which is initially firmly closed and shows a dynamic relaxation in response to buttock separation.**

6.46   There is no doubt that reflex anal dilatation is commoner in anally abused children than in any other group. However the reported incidence fluctuates substantially from investigator to investigator and this may reflect differences in technique, degree of reassurance, degree of traction applied and anxiety on the part of the child rather than any intrinsic differences in interpretation of similar physical findings. These many variables may explain those instances where RAD has fluctuated in the same child from one day to another.

Summary of perianal signs in abuse

6.47   It is of the utmost importance that examination techniques are standardised and that such variables as the degree of dilatation in millimetres, the persistence, reproducibility and, if possible, length of time to disappearance of the sign be recorded. **The Working Party is agreed that the occurrence of reflex anal dilatation which is reproducible in an otherwise normal child would be a cause for concern, justifying follow-up. This concern would increase in the presence of additional anal signs, eg fresh fissures, especially outside the midline.**

6.48   It is obvious from the evidence set out in this chapter that no clear statements can be made as to the significance of physical findings in the anal region in individual cases, with the exception of major lacerations or scar (para 6.49(1)).

6.49   Perianal signs may be summarised as follows:

1. Diagnostic of blunt force penetrating trauma. The only absolute indicator of anal abuse is a laceration or a healed scar extending beyond the anal mucosa onto the perianal skin in the absence of reasonable alternative explanation, eg major trauma. Scars are seen in only a small proportion (less than 10%) of children with positive anal findings.

2. Supportive but not diagnostic.

a   anal laxity without other explanation.

b   reflex anal dilatation greater than 1 cm.

c   acute changes, eg erythema, swelling, fissures, venous congestion and bruising. These are thought to be seen more frequently in the 0–5-year age group.

d   chronic changes, eg 'funnelling' in chronic abuse in older children; the triad of signs of frequent anal intercourse,[15] ie (a) thickness of the anal verge skin—with resultant reduction in anal verge skin folds, (b) increased elasticity, and (c) reduction in power of the anal sphincter.

3. There may be no discernible physical changes at the anus despite the practice of abuse.

4. The Working Party notes the US view (oral evidence) that RAD greater than 2 cm indicates penetrating trauma. The view of the Working Party is that this finding—in the absence of alternative explanation— is **more likely than not to be associated with abuse**. This likelihood increases if the sign is reproducible and associated with other consistent features.

7 Association of physical with sexual abuse

7.1   There is an association between different types of abuse, and a diagnosis of any form of abuse indicates that a medical assessment for sexual abuse should be considered.

7.2   About 15% of sexually abused children have been violently abused. One hundred and thirty children are reported[34] with appearance of both physical and sexual abuse. Bruises in physical abuse alone are often on the head, neck and back but in sexual abuse significant bruising is around the knees, thighs and genitalia. Grip marks showing 4 or 5 finger tips down the thighs, and symmetrical bruises around the knees are highly suggestive of sexual abuse with forceful gripping by the abuser. Burns may also be seen on the buttocks, thighs and lower abdomen. Other injuries include bite marks, particularly on the breasts, lower abdomen, buttocks or genitalia, 'love bites' and signs of trauma inside the mouth.

8 Healing of physical signs

8.1   Healing may occur within hours or days, or may take weeks or months depending on the severity and chronicity. Fresh erythema, abrasions and bruises will fade within a few days.

8.2   A single episode of anal abuse may result in perianal swelling, a gaping anus and reflex dilatation, which may clear within 7–10 days.

8.3   Chronic abuse is likely to lead to changes of much longer duration and any scars will probably be permanent.

8.4   Reflex anal dilatation may cease within one to six weeks, but in some children the dilatation can still be elicited many months after the abuse has ceased.[21]

8.5   Deep anal fissures may take months to heal, and distended perianal veins may be one of the last signs to fade. In the vast majority of abused children eventual healing will be almost complete in the perianal region.

8.6   Healing of hymenal injuries may be very rapid. From studies of acute trauma, such as a laceration or tear, it is known that the hymen may heal completely within 2 weeks after a single episode. Sometimes the healing process may result in considerable scarring and leave a small contracted hymenal opening. All that can be deduced therefore from a hymenal opening of, for example, 5 mm with scarring is that there has been no penetration within the previous 2 weeks. It has also been reported[35] that follow-up examination 2 years after documented trauma has shown in some instances that the hymenal diameter had returned to normal.

When penetration is repeated, the hymen does not recover its original form.

9 Forensic evidence

Procedures

9.1   When medical evaluation is being carried out for suspected sexual abuse it is of the utmost importance that correct procedures are followed for the collection of evidential material and forensic samples.

9.2   Ideally, joint examinations by police surgeons and paediatricians ensure that the forensic aspects are properly dealt with. However, in recent years there has been an increasing number of referrals to paediatricians for suspected sexual abuse and a joint examination is not always practicable. Hence, paediatricians and other doctors undertaking such work should be familiar with relevant forensic procedures and should have access to 'rape kits', ie the standard boxes of sample containers, plastic bags and labels kept by most police sexual abuse units. It is also necessary for the doctor to make detailed records, including word-for-word reports of conversations with the child, prepare reports, attend case conferences and give evidence in court if necessary. These aspects have implications for training.

9.3   In some areas, the Area Child Protection Committee (ACPC) has recommended a suitable proforma should be completed as part of the collection of forensic evidence. Doctors should be aware of local forensic practices.

Chain of evidence

9.4   The principle of the Chain of Evidence must be recognised and its importance appreciated with regard to all samples which may ultimately be used for evidential purposes.
    The Chain of Evidence is a legal concept which requires that **the origin and history of any exhibit to be presented as evidence in a Court of Law must be clearly demonstrated to have followed an unbroken chain from its source to the Court.** All persons handling the sample and the places and conditions of storage must be documented, with a note of the time, date and place and signatures where appropriate.
    Some cases will involve the presentation of the actual exhibit in court but more commonly, for example for swabs and other biological specimens, the report is acceptable if the chain to the report can be shown to be intact.

Problems arise when the need to start a formal chain is not appreciated. A swab initially intended for clinical purposes may show the presence of a sexually transmitted disease which may be of important evidential value. **Unless the chain of evidence has been initiated by the physician, the result will be inadmissible in court.**

A chain involving a swab in a case of suspected sexual abuse may involve the physician taking the swab, the police officer or laboratory technician to whom it is handed, the technician dealing with and examining the swab and the forensic scientist or microbiologist. The physician taking the swab must seal it, label it fully and hand it to the next person in the chain, noting the date, time and person to whom it is handed.

9.5   In cases of alleged chronic abuse, when the last episode was more than a week before the investigation, evidence collection consists of a careful history and physical examination, as well as taking samples for examination for sexually transmitted diseases.

9.6   When the last contact or acute assault has been within 72 hours, forensic evidence should always be sought using as far as possible the techniques used in adult rape cases. With appropriate samples and forensic analysis, it may be possible to establish that abuse did take place and that the perpetrator ejaculated. On occasion it is possible to confirm the identity of a perpetrator using DNA techniques.

9.7   The time limits for detection of spermatozoa are 12 to 14 hours for oral samples, 6 days for vaginal samples and 3 days for anal swabs. The time limits for detection of seminal fluid are 12–18 hours in the vagina and 3 hours in the anus.

9.8   In the case of recent assault, it is advisable to arrange for a police representative to be available to receive the samples, clothing etc. The child is undressed on a spread sheet of clean paper in order to collect any loose particles caught up in the clothing. Stained items and underclothes should be placed in the bags provided and labelled with the date, time and names of the patient and the examiner.

9.9   The skin should be inspected for any stains or loose hairs. The presence of semen which has dried on the body can be demonstrated by a Wood's lamp which causes the semen to fluoresce a green colour. If the hair is matted with semen, a sample should be cut off. The fluorescence of semen should be easily distinguished from the brilliant white patches in the skin, shown by a Wood's lamp, in some neurocutaneous disorders and from some detergents and other preparations.

9.10   Swabs should be taken as appropriate:

  i Skin swabs for lubricant, semen, saliva.

 ii Circum and intra-oral swabs, in particular from the labial-gingival fold for spermatozoa.

iii External vaginal swab.

iv Internal vaginal swab if hymenal orifice allows when relaxed.

 v External anal swab.

vi Internal anal swab.

The swabs may be dampened with water but *not* with grease.

Screening for STD

9.11   Swabs must also be taken for sexually transmitted diseases (STD). In the case of young children, especially if frightened by recent abuse, it may be impossible to persuade the child to allow the optimal number of swabs to be taken and discretion is required as to the more important samples in each individual case.

9.12   In Appendix 2, a flow chart is provided which incorporates both forensic and STD samples for screening. Appendix 3 gives detailed guidance on forensic samples.

DNA techniques

9.13   It is unusual to try to identify the perpetrator by the use of forensic samples but this aspect may become more important as DNA techniques become more freely available. Most of the genetic markers present in blood are also present in semen. ABO blood group antigens, and the enzyme markers phosphoglucomutase (PGM) and peptidase-A (pep A) are present in semen in high enough concentrations for typing for evidential purposes. However, the blood group antigens are secreted into body fluids by only 80% of the population. This secretor status can be tested in a sample of saliva. Combined ABO and PGM subtyping, when possible, allows for genetic differentiation in about 90% of cases.

9.14   Blood or semen stains are best preserved by rapid drying and frozen storage. If suitably dried, immediately after collection, genetic markers can be typed for weeks and, if frozen, for months or years. PGM is helpful only if the swabs are collected within 6 hours of intercourse, and pep A within 3 hours.

10 Sexually transmitted disease in child abuse (See also Appendix 4)

Significance of positive findings

10.1   It is recognised that a small proportion of sexually abused children have sexually transmitted disease (STD). The question arises as to whether evidence of STD is, of itself, evidence of sexual abuse. It is unsafe to regard STD as being exclusively sexually transmitted. There are no documented cases of transmission by fomites but there are cases of apparent asexual transmission person-to-person in the case of herpes simplex, syphilis[36] and gonorrhoea. In addition, transmission from mother to infant perinatally is well documented for most STDs and some, eg human papilloma virus and *Chlamydia trachomatis*, may lie dormant for some time.

10.2   If the presence of STD is to be used for evidential purposes, the importance of the 'chain of evidence' is emphasised.

10.3   Sexually transmitted disease, occurring after infancy in children and adolescents who are not sexually active is strongly suggestive but not proof of sexual abuse. Gonorrhoea is presumptive evidence of sexual contact.[7,37]

10.4   Since many of these infections may remain asymptomatic for a period, it is important to screen children suspected of having been sexually abused.

10.5   When other indicators of sexual abuse exist and a child is also found to have a sexually transmitted disease, then the diagnosis of abuse is virtually certain.

Treatment in acute abuse

10.6   With regard to emergency treatment for possible infection, there is controversy about the indications for prophylaxis with antibiotics. It was suggested from data based on adult women[38] (1971) that in acute abuse the rate for acquisition of gonorrhoea was 3.5% and of syphilis 0.2%. The incidence of chlamydial infection has not been studied. Appropriate cultures should be obtained and close follow-up care given so that treatment may be instituted if indicated.

10.7   There is a case to be made for giving prophylactic treatment
following on acute assault as part of the psychological healing process.[7]
It is however not routinely recommended. Indications for treatment
would be: first psychological; second, when there is real concern about
STD; and last, if facilities are not available for appropriate culture.

11 Prophylaxis against pregnancy

11.1   Post-coital pregnancy prophylaxis should be offered to post-menarchal girls (if not already pregnant) presenting within 72 hours of an acute episode of abuse. Those presenting later should be closely monitored in case of developing pregnancy. It is the duty of the doctor who receives the relevant information to arrange for such treatment to be given. The estimated incidence of pregnancy following abuse is low, about 1% in a random sample, rising to 10% if the assault occurred mid-cycle.[7]

Summary and conclusions

1. A substantial proportion of sexually abused children show no abnormal physical findings (para 4.12).

2. There are as yet insufficient data on the range and variation in appearances of the normal pre-pubertal male and female genitalia, based upon a population of children who have not been abused. Establishing that the children have not been abused raises ethical considerations which make such data difficult to obtain.

3. Physical findings are influenced by the examination techniques employed.

It is recommended that the female genitalia are normally examined in the supine frog-legged position, using labial separation and gentle labial traction to display the hymenal orifice (paras 2.13, 2.14). Some doctors experienced in the field have used in addition the knee–elbow position, which may yield additional information (para 2.11).

The anus is examined in the left lateral position with hips and knees well flexed. The buttocks are gently separated and the anal sphincter observed for 30 seconds (para 2.17).

4. There are a number of anatomical variations in the normal child, for example bumps or notches on the hymen, which may also appear in a modified form in abuse (paras 3.9, 3.10).

5. Non-specific signs which occur in abused children may also be seen in non-abused children, for example inflammation, superficial fissures of the posterior fourchette and perineum, fusion of the labia minora and vaginal discharge. Poor hygiene and scratching are contributory factors (para 4.10).

6. The hymenal orifice dimension is not a reliable indicator of sexual abuse, although a horizontal diameter exceeding 1 cm in a pre-pubertal child occurs more commonly in abused girls. It is a feature which should arouse suspicion (para 4.5).

7. Very few signs are diagnostic of abuse in the absence of reasonable alternative explanation. These are a laceration or scar of the hymen, attenuation of the hymen with loss of hymenal tissue (para 4.14) and a laceration or scar of the anal mucosa extending beyond the anal verge onto the perianal skin (para 6.49). Pregnancy in a child or young person under 16 years of age should raise the question of abuse.

8. There is a clear overlap between abused and non-abused populations with regard to physical signs which are consistent with and even suggestive of abuse. This is particularly so in the case of anal findings and reflex anal dilatation (para 6.38).

There is no doubt that a substantial proportion of children subjected to anal abuse show dilatation of the anal canal on buttock separation while most non-abused children do not. However, reflex anal dilatation cannot by itself be regarded as an indication of abuse in the individual case, although it is a sign which supports a child's story of abuse.

9. Gross anal dilatation which is persistent, reproducible and greater than 1.5 cm diameter is probably more significant than lesser degrees of dilatation.

10. The diagnosis of child sexual abuse is confirmed following a multi-disciplinary investigation with full inter-agency cooperation (para 6.3). Physical findings—including normality—are consistent with abuse and it is therefore important to document carefully even minor ano-genital signs as well as negative findings. The single most important feature is a statement by the child. Detailed medical and forensic evidence may support this statement, as may a psychological assessment of the child or the confession by a perpetrator.

Physical signs alone are on rare occasions sufficient to make the diagnosis. The interpretation of physical findings is a matter for a doctor with experience in this field (para 2.3). A multi-disciplinary investigation with full inter-agency cooperation is necessary whenever there is concern that child sexual abuse has occurred.

References

1. *Report of the inquiry into child abuse in Cleveland.* HMSO, 1987: 247.
2. Tipton A. Child sexual abuse: physical examination techniques and interpretation of findings. *Adolesc Pediatr Gynecol* 1989; **2**: 10–25.
3. *Report of the inquiry into child abuse in Cleveland.* HMSO, 1987: 184.
4. Woodling B, Heger A. The use of the colposcope in the diagnosis of sexual abuse. *Child Abuse Negl* 1986; **10**: 111–4.
5. Jenny C, Kuhns M, Arakawa F. Hymens in newborn female infants. *Pediatrics* 1987; **80**: 399–400.
6. Pokorny S. Configuration of the prepubertal hymen. *Am J Obstet Gynecol* 1987; **157**: 950–6.
7. Berkowitz C. Sexual abuse of children and adolescents. Chapter in *Adv Pediatr* 1987; **34**: 275–312.
8. Handfield-Jones S, Hinde F, Kennedy C. Lichen sclerosus et atrophicus in children misdiagnosed as sexual abuse. *Br Med J* 1987; **294**: 1404–5.
9. Priestley B, Bleehen S. Lichen sclerosus and sexual abuse. *Arch Dis Child* 1990; **65**: 335.
10. Pokorny S, Kozinetz C. Configuration and other anatomic details of the prepubertal hymen. *Adolesc Pediatr Gynecol* 1988; **1**: 97–103.
11. Muram D. Child sexual abuse: relationship between sexual acts and genital findings. *Child Abuse Negl* 1989; **13**: 211–6.
12. Cantwell J. Vaginal inspection as it relates to child sexual abuse in girls under 13. *Child Abuse Negl* 1983; **7**: 171–6.
13. White S, Ingram D. Vaginal introital diameter in the evaluation of sexual abuse. *Child Abuse Negl* 1989; **13**: 217–24.
14. Woodling B. Sexual abuse and the child. *Em Med Serv* 1986; **15**: 17–25.
15. Muram D. Child sexual abuse: genital tract findings in prepubertal girls. *Am J Obstet Gynecol* 1989; **160**: 328–33.
16. Paul D. The medical aspects of alleged sexual abuse of children. *Med Sci Law* 1986; **26**: 85–102.
17. Paradise J, Willis E. Probability of vaginal foreign body in girls with genital complaints. *Am J Dis Child* 1985; **139**: 472–6.
18. Woodling B, Kossoris P. Sexual misuse. *Pediatr Clin North Am* 1981; **28**(2): 481–500.
19. DHSS. *Working together.* HMSO, 1988.
20. Krugman R. Editorial. *Child Abuse Negl* 1989; **13**: 165–6.
21. Hobbs C, Wynne J. Sexual abuse of English boys and girls: the importance of anal examination. *Child Abuse Negl* 1989; **13**: 195–210.
22. McCann J, Voris J, Simon M, Wells R. Perianal findings in prepubertal children selected for non-abuse. *Child Abuse Negl* 1989; **13**: 179–93.
23. Lanktree C, Zaidi L, Briere J, Gutterez V. Differential identification of sexually abused children in psychiatric outpatients. Abstract. *Amer Psychological Assoc*, New Orleans. August 1989.
24. Agnarsson U, Gordon C, Wright C, *et al.* Perianal appearances in childhood constipation. *Arch Dis Child* 1990; **65**: 1231–4.
25. Melzak J, Porter N. Studies of the reflex activity of the external sphincter ani in spinal man. *Paraplegia* 1960; **1**: 277–96.
26. Goligher J. *Surgery of the anus, rectum and colon,* Baillière Tindall, 1984.
27. Allen-Mersh T. Evidence presented to Working Party.
28. Hobbs C, Wynne J. Buggery in childhood. *Lancet* 1986; **ii**: 792–6.
29. Wright C, Fraser E, Denman M, Duke L. Detection of sexual abuse in children. *Lancet* 1987; **ii**: 218.
30. Stanton A, Sunderland R. Prevalence of reflex anal dilatation in 200 children. *Br Med J* 1989; **298**: 802–3.

31. Priestley B. Reflex anal dilatation and abuse. *Lancet* 1987; **ii**: 1396.
32. Clayden G. Reflex anal dilatation associated with severe chronic constipation in children. *Arch Dis Child* 1988; **63**: 832–6.
33. Kirschner R, Stein R. The mistaken diagnosis of child abuse. *Am J Dis Child* 1985; **139**: 873–5.
34. Hobbs CJ and Wynne JM. The sexually abused battered child. *Arch Dis Child* 1990; **65**: 423–427.
35. Cantwell J. Update on vaginal inspection. *Child Abuse Negl* 1987; **11**: 545–6.
36. Neinstein L, Goldenring J, Carpenter S. Non-sexual transmission of sexually transmitted diseases: an infrequent occurrence. *Pediatrics* 1984; **74**: 67–76.
37. Glaser J, Hammerschlag M, McCormack W. Sexually transmitted disease in victims of sexual assault. *N Engl J Med* 1986; **315**: 625–7.
38. Hayman C, Lanza C. Sexual assault on women and girls. *Am J Obstet Gynecol* 1971; **109**: 480–6.

APPENDIX 1

Glossary of terms — anal signs

Anal canal folds Because the anus is required to expand to allow passage of a formed stool, both the epithelial lining of the anal canal, and the skin of the anal verge exhibit regular folds when the anus is closed. In the anal canal, the epithelial folds are vertical along the length of the canal, are most prominent in the upper half of the canal and extend into the lower few centimetres of the rectum proper. These folds can be thickened by regular trauma, eg repeated sodomy, and the epithelium may undergo squamous metaplasia, causing the folds both to look and to feel calloused. If the anal tissues become swollen (as a result of oedema or bruising) the folds become less obvious or may even disappear.

It is important to distinguish between anal canal folds when the skin is intact, and fissures, when there is a break in continuity.

Anal fissure An anal fissure consists of a crack in the skin-lined part of the anal canal. Fissures may be single or multiple (fissuring). *Acute fissure*: this is a superficial fissure with only the skin cracked. *Chronic fissure*: this is a deep fissure — the transverse fibres of the internal sphincter are seen in the base.

Anal twitching ('winking') Brief recurrent visible contractions of the external anal sphincter. External sphincter contraction cannot be sustained, and where voluntary effort is being made to maintain anal closure, anal twitching or winking may occur in the absence of external stimulation. It has been observed in anally abused children and may draw attention to the possibility of abuse. Caution in interpreting the significance of the sign is necessary because the frequency of its occurrence in circumstances other than abuse is unknown. At most, it is weak corroborative evidence of abuse.

Anal verge defect This is an indentation in the anal verge but lined throughout by unbroken skin. In normal children, such areas are in the *midline*, either anteriorly or posteriorly, and represent a gap in the fibres of the corrugator cutis ani muscle, ie the superficial part of the external sphincter. The significance of *lateral* verge defects is unclear, but their origin must be different since the external sphincter is not deficient laterally.

Constipation The definition of a normal bowel habit is 'the passage of a formed stool once daily'. However, in children wide variation of this norm is common and anything from three or four bowel actions daily to one bowel action every third day is within the range of normality, provided that the stool consistency is normal and the act of defaecation untroubled. Minor or occasional deviations from this range are of little significance. When a child regularly has a bowel habit outside the normal range or has symptoms and the rectum is loaded, then significant constipation is present.

In this case, the loaded rectum is not completely emptied by a normal defaecation effort and an exaggerated effort (straining) is required. Some children habitually strain to defaecate and this may occur even in the presence of an empty rectum; since this effort is not attended by the passage of a stool, the child may incorrectly be described as 'constipated'.

Eversion of the anal canal   This is very rarely observed, and is usually associated with a rectal prolapse. This is often the result of anatomical features that are unrelated to anal penetration, eg weak pelvic floor, absence of the normal sacral curve, or spinal cord maldevelopment. Very severe trauma to the pelvic floor and sphincter muscles could cause an eversion but would be associated with evidence of such injury.

Friability of perianal skin   The perianal skin is moistened, presumably by an increase in mucus discharged from the anus, which leads to fissuring or friability of the soggy perianal skin. Similar changes may occur with excessive sweating, obesity, eczema and in association with other changes in lichen sclerosis.

Funnelled anus   Some children are born with an anal canal that does not close at rest in its lowest 1–2 cm. In these children the anal canal, when viewed from the perineal aspect, does not have the usual tubular shape but funnels down from the open anal verge to its closed upper lumen. Because of this appearance, this condition is known as 'the funnelled anus'.

In older forensic texts, this term was used to describe a funnelled approach to the anal canal, in association with obliteration of fatty tissue consequent upon chronic anal intercourse. It is doubtful whether the condition exists.

Gaping or patulous anus   A floppy irregular opening of the anus arising from paralysis of the anal sphincter. It may occur in children with neuro-muscular disorders, especially in paraplegic children, eg in myelomeningocoele and those with sacral agenesis. These neurological disorders need to be considered in the differential diagnosis of anal abuse.

Haematoma of anal margin   This refers to bruising in or beneath the skin at the anal verge. It may be caused by a penetrative act of abuse, resulting in shearing of the subcutaneous venous plexus and haematoma formation.

Hypertrophied anal papilla   The anal valve at the proximal end of an anal fold may become oedematous and inflamed, which may result in thickening. The cause is uncertain.

Lax sphincter   A lax sphincter is one that has a lower than normal level of anal tone. In the absence of anal manometry, the assessment of anal tone is achieved by digital insertion. Although such observation of anal tone is wholly subjective it is surprisingly accurate when a comparison is made between digital 'impression' and manometric measurement. A lax anus often gapes and such gaping may be made more obvious by buttock retraction. Diminished external anal sphincter tone is mainly responsible for a lax sphincter muscle; the internal anal sphincter is often normal in such patients.

A lax sphincter may lack the usual responses to stimulation. Therefore the ano-rectal reflex may be absent, and augmentation of anal sphincter tone on coughing may not be present.

A lax anus may be seen in a normal infant or toddler, in patients under general anaesthesia and in some critically ill children. It is also found in association with severe constipation, ie hard faecal masses in an abnormally distended rectum (megarectum); in patients with a patulous anus of neurogenic origin, and in association with anal abuse.

Perianal pigmentation and lichenification Irregular thickening of peri-anal skin and a greater degree of pigmentation than in surrounding skin. It may be a consequence of any long continued abrasion of the skin surface. Scratching is common in childhood. There are several innocent causes of perianal pigmentation and lichenification including eczema and lichen sclerosus et atrophicus. Caution is needed in interpreting hyperpigmentation in children of non-European racial origin. It is not reliable as an isolated sign but in the context of abuse, recurrent abuse is implied.

Perianal venous dilatation This refers to a skin-covered collection of veins at the perianal region which is usually crescentic but may encircle the anus. It may be a normal finding in babies who are observed to be straining as at defaecation. The distended normal veins are part of the external haemorrhoidal plexus. They fade when defaecation has been completed. Persistence of venous dilatation extending beyond the anal verge is sometimes found in association with anal abuse.

Reflex anal dilatation The physiological explanation for this reaction is unclear. Opening of the anus after a brief period of buttock separation arises from weakness or relaxation of the external anal sphincter accompanied by relaxation of the internal sphincter. Distension of the lower rectum may cause reflex relaxation of the internal anal sphincter and the sign may be seen in children who have a loaded rectum or who are straining. In a relaxed child who has an empty rectum, it may be indicative of trauma to the anal sphincter and should draw attention to the possibility of anal abuse, but as an isolated sign it is not pathognomonic of abuse. Minor degrees of relaxation should be disregarded, ie less than 0.5 cm to 1 cm.

Sentinel 'pile' or skin tag This is a result of inflammatory reaction and oedema at the lower end of a fissure—it may be acute or undergo fibrosis and become permanent.

Tyre sign Prominence of a ring of tissue surrounding the anal orifice giving it the appearance of a tyre. It has been described in sexually abused children but whether or not it occurs in other conditions is not known, nor is it known how long the sign persists after the cessation of abuse. Theoretically, the prominence may be due to external anal sphincter hypertrophy, tissue oedema or simply an anatomical variant. The first two may have implications with

respect to anal abuse but the sign in isolation is not diagnostic. It may draw
attention to the possibility of abuse and provide weak corroborative evidence.

Visibly relaxed sphincter   A visual impression of diminished anal sphincter
tone arising from reduced puckering of the perianal skin and possibly slight
opening of the anus. It may occur following long continued receptive anal
intercourse but in the context of child sexual abuse it is of doubtful significance.
It may also occur in chronic constipation.

APPENDIX 2

An outline approach to medical and forensic investigation of child sexual abuse

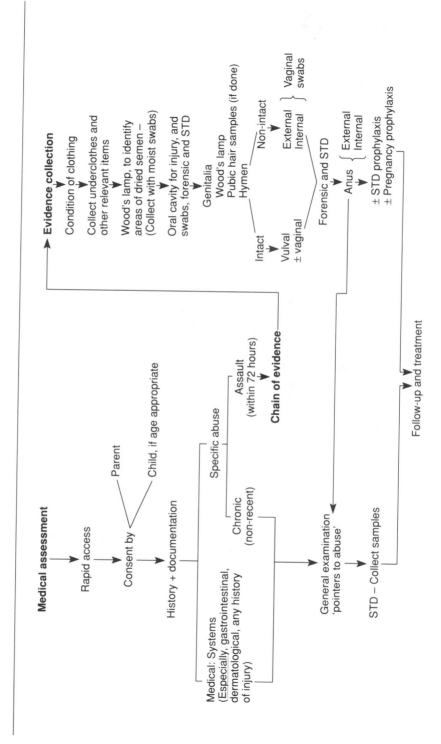

APPENDIX 3a

Prepared by: Dr D. Jenkins, Dr F. Lewington
Metropolitan Police Forensic Science Laboratory

The significance of forensic medical samples which may be taken in suspected child sexual abuse

1.   These comments and the information given in Appendix 3b refer to samples which may be taken in cases of chronic child sexual abuse where there may have been a recent assault; samples needed to investigate the identity of the perpetrator are not included.

2.   The forensic samples fall into two categories:

   a evidential samples;

   b control samples (blood and saliva) for comparison purposes.

3.   These samples will be examined in a Forensic Science Laboratory. It is most important that the recommended sampling materials and containers are used and that the precise storage instructions are followed, so that the maximum information is obtained. The sampling materials and instructions are usually supplied in kit form by individual police forces.

4.   The scientific examination is based primarily on 'Locard's Principle' that 'every contact leaves a trace'.[1] The evidential trace materials fall into two types: (i) those which occur as loose debris or particles, and (ii) those which occur as stains. The evidential samples taken at the medical examination involve the use of plain cotton wool swabs to remove evidentially important stains, and the use of forceps or swabs to remove particulate debris. If stains are dry, swabs can be moistened with distilled water (or tap water) but not saline.

5.   The evidential trace materials which are most likely to be important in child sexual abuse examinations are:

Stains		*Debris*
Blood	Lubricants	Pubic hair
Semen	Faeces	
Saliva		
Vaginal fluid		

Materials such as textile fibres, head hairs and fragments of wood, paint, glass etc are unlikely to be evidentially important where the perpetrator is a member of the same household or extended family of the victim.

6.   The scientific examination may also concern the analysis of preserved blood and urine samples for alcohol, drugs and solvents.

7.   Unless the abuse occurred recently (see 8 below), samples taken at the medical examination are less likely to yield useful evidence than unwashed clothing, bedding, carpets, sofa covers and items used in the assault, such as a stick or a bottle neck, examined for blood, semen, saliva, vaginal fluid, faeces, lubricants etc.

8.   *Time limits for the detection of spermatozoa and seminal fluid*:

	Spermatozoa	*Seminal fluid*
Vagina	6 days[2]	12–18 hours[2]
Anus	3 days[3]	3 hours[4]
Mouth	12–14 hours[5]	—
Clothing/bedding	until washed	until washed

At present, no similar figures are available for the likely retrieval of other evidential material from the body.

9.   *Labelling and sealing*:

i Individual bags, bottles and swabs should be labelled with:

   a   name of patient;

   b   date taken;

   c   person taking sample;

   d   type of sample.

ii In addition, a 'Criminal Justice Act' label must be attached to the container or the outer wrapping. This label has spaces for the type of sample and sample number to be entered, and the signatures of the producer of the sample and all who handle the sample until it is produced in court. Individual sample numbers are formed using the producer's initials and starting with 1 for the first sample taken, eg *ABC/1 Saliva sample, ABC/2 Urine sample*. For each new examination, the doctor will start again at 1, except where two or more children are examined as part of the same inquiry, when the numbers will follow consecutively, eg *ABC/1–10* for samples taken from the older child and *ABC/11–20* for samples taken from her sister.

iii All samples must be sealed with clear adhesive tape over a signed 'signature' label. Freezer tape should be used for blood, urine and saliva bottles, swabs and any other items to be refrigerated or frozen. The tape must be wound completely around the neck of bottles and swab caps over the signature label. When sealing bags, the top of the bag should be turned over at least

2.5 cm, turned over again, fastened down with the signature label followed by a strip of adhesive tape which is sufficiently long for the free ends to be fastened to the reverse of the bag.

iv Many police forces, including the Metropolitan Police, are introducing specially manufactured sample bags which incorporate the 'Criminal Justice Label' and signature label in the self-adhesive flap of the bag.

10. *Samples for sexually transmitted diseases testing*

These samples will not be examined in the Forensic Science Laboratory, and for each area individual arrangements will need to be made with the local hospital services. In 'stranger' attacks, the STD samples will need to be taken separately from the 'forensic' samples after an appropriate incubation period and may need to be repeated. In cases of chronic abuse, the local arrangements should be confirmed at the planning stage of the medical examination, as in some hospitals these samples will be taken by the forensic medical examiner whereas in other areas a doctor from the special clinic will attend to take the samples, or arrangements will be made for the patient to attend the clinic for a private appointment.

The materials for these samples are not provided in the 'police kits' and arrangements will need to be made for local hospital supplies to be available.

References

1. Locard E. Dust and its analysis. *Police Journal* 1928; **1**: 177–92.
2. Davies A, Wilson EM. The persistence of seminal constituents in the human vagina. *Forensic Science* 1974; **3**: 45–55.
3. Willott GM, Allard JE. Spermatozoa and their persistence after sexual intercourse. *Forensic Science International* 1982; **19**: 135–54.
4. Metropolitan Police Forensic Science Laboratory, unpublished.
5. Willcott GM, Crosse MM. The detection of spermatozoa in the mouth. *Journal of the Forensic Science Society* 1986; **26**: 125–8.

APPENDIX 3b

Forensic medical samples: check list and guidelines

Samples	Examination	Sampling materials, Packing/Containers	Comments
1. *Clothing* (if thought to have been worn during the assault)	Damage; stain location and identification; pubic hairs	Paper bags for dry clothing; open polythene bags for wet items	
2. *Urine* (routine sample)	Drug/alcohol assay	Bottle containing sodium fluoride	Extra tact may be required if child was made to urinate as part of sexual act
3. *Blood* (5 ml)	Alcohol/drugs/solvent assay	Bottle containing sodium fluoride and potassium oxalate	In addition to date on sample bottle, record time taken.
4. *Saliva*	Detection of semen	Bottle without additive	Difficult to obtain. Recommend that the child is given the bottle at the start of the medical examination to leave as much time as possible to obtain sample
5. *Mouth swab*	Detection of semen	Plain sterile swabs	More likely to detect semen in saliva sample than on mouth swab
6. *Skin swabs*	Detection of lubricants, blood, semen and saliva	Plain sterile swabs	If stain is dry, the swab should be moistened with tap water, not saliva

7. *External vaginal swab*	Detection of lubricants, blood, semen, saliva	Plain sterile swabs	External swab to be taken before internal. Swabs can be dampened with water. Grease should not be used. In pre-pubertal children, internal swabs should only be taken when abuse has involved obvious penetration
8. *Internal vaginal swab*			
9. *External anal swab*	Detection of blood, semen, saliva and lubricants	Plain sterile swabs	External swab to be taken before internal. Swabs can be dampened with water. Grease should not be used. Both swabs should be considered *even* if there is no obvious injury to the anus
10. *Internal anal swab*			
11. *Penile swab* (swabbing from outside of penis)	For semen, saliva, lubricants	Plain sterile swab	Urethral swabs are not required
12. *Matted head hair*	Semen	Polythene bag	Matted area is cut out
13. *Loose pubic hairs*	Identification of alien hairs	Polythene bags	
14. *Pubic hairs* (combed)*	Retrieval of possible alien hairs	Polythene bags	Leave hairs on comb, return to bag
15. *Pubic hairs—cut* *	Control sample for comparison with alien hairs	Polythene bags	10–25 hairs if possible cut next to skin
16. *Matted pubic hair*	Semen	Polythene bags	Matted area is cut out

*The Metropolitan Police Laboratories no longer include these items in their procedure because of possible discomfort to the child and because improved DNA testing facilities make it unnecessary.

APPENDIX 4a

Sexually transmitted diseases in child abuse

Introduction

Non-sexual transmission of sexually transmitted disease(s) (STD) is rarely an issue in adults. When STD occur in children sexual abuse must be suspected. However some STD have a long and variable latent period and there are reports of other non-sexual methods of transmission, albeit infrequently. This makes it difficult to use the presence of STD as an absolute indication that abuse has taken place. It may be used as corroborative evidence. In some cases, for example when the same STD is identified in the alleged assailant and the child and other sources of infection have been excluded (eg perinatally acquired from the mother), it may be conclusive evidence that abuse has taken place.

The following report is a brief summary of STD for the non-specialist; it excludes treatment and draws attention to pitfalls in diagnosis. The diagnostic ability of the microbiology/virology departments is dependent upon the quality of the specimens received. It is therefore advisable that these should be taken by an appropriately trained person, usually a paediatrician or GU physician, depending on local arrangements.

Departments of Genitourinary Medicine may be able to offer training and in liaison with the pathology departments ensure that the appropriate specimen bottles and swabs are available.

Appendix 4b provides a simple guide to specimen taking and diagnosis. The presence of one STD indicates the need to look for others and in cases of suspected child sexual abuse it is advisable to screen for STD even in the absence of symptoms.

Gonorrhoea

Neisseria gonorrhoeae is a Gram negative intracellular diplococcus which primarily infects columnar or transitional epithelium.

A presumptive identification of *N. gonorrhoeae* in a Gram-stain smear can be used as a guide, but the diagnosis depends upon culture of the organism on a gonococcal selective medium (Thayer Martin) with 5% CO_2 at 37°C, and is confirmed by either carbohydrate degradation tests, enzyme substrate tests or immunological tests. Insufficient characterisation of Neisseria species may result in incorrect diagnosis and has resulted in false allegations of abuse.[1]

N. gonorrhoeae requires intimate contact with epithelial or mucus secreting cells for transmission. Infection may occur in the urethra, endocervix, conjunctiva, oropharynx, prepubertal vagina and rectum. Cultures should be obtained from multiple sites from children who are suspected of being abused. The incubation period is from 3 to 7 days. Infection may be asymptomatic, particularly pharyngeal infection.[2] De Jong[3] found 56% of infected children had symptoms which included vaginal or rectal discharge and rectal discomfort.

The frequency of infection with *N. gonorrhoeae* in studies of sexually abused children presenting to sexual assault centres ranges from 2.3%[3] to 11.2%[4] and is more likely with multiple episodes of abuse.[3]

The question arises as to the possibility of gonorrhoea in children being transmitted through close non-sexual contact or close contact with infected underwear or linen. The gonococcus has been shown to survive on toilet seats for 2 to 24 hours[6,7] and as long as 72 hours on other materials, eg wooden spatula, cardboard, charcoal dipped cotton swab.[8] Acquisition of gonorrhoea by non-sexual means is not thought to occur in adults and reports on non-sexual transmission in children stress over-crowded living conditions. Others have not specifically addressed the question of sexual abuse. However, it has not proved possible to attribute all cases conclusively to sexual abuse in any of the larger published series.[9,10]

In children less than one year of age, infection is usually the result of ocular contamination through maternal-child transmission.[11]

Studies from 1976 onwards have considered the possibility of sexual contact or abuse more closely. The bulk of evidence suggests that gonorrhoea in children is a sexually transmitted disease and the isolation of a gonococcal infection is highly suggestive of abuse.

Chlamydia trachomatis (CT)

CT organisms are obligate intracellular bacteria with a unique developmental cycle involving an infectious extracellular form (elementary body) which attaches to the host cell (columnar or transitional epithelium), enters by endocytosis and differentiates into a non-infectious intracellular form (reticulate body). After approximately 36 hours the reticulate bodies differentiate into elementary bodies which are released at about 48 hours. As a result of this life cycle, there may be prolonged subclinical infection which is a hallmark of human chlamydial disease.

Disease is subdivided into ocular (trachoma) and genital forms associated with different serotypes of CT. Lymphogranuloma venereum (LGV) is a tropical STD caused by CT serotypes L1, L2 and L3 which are antigenically and biologically different from oculogenital strains.

Diagnosis of CT

Methods include culture, enzyme immunoassay (EIA) and direct immuno-fluorescent (IF) antibody test (eg MicroTrak). Culture remains the 'gold' standard but is not widely available because it requires special handling of specimens and cell culture technique.

It is important when taking specimens to use cotton tipped swabs and to remove the swab from the bottle as some materials, eg wood are toxic to the cell culture. Although the EIA and IF methods have been extensively evaluated for genital specimens from adults, few studies have been done in paediatric populations.

EIA tests for *Chlamydia* detect the presence of lipopolysaccharide antigen and not viable organisms. It may cross react with other bacterial antigens giving false positive signals. False positive results from rectal swabs have been reported in children.[12] Hammerschlag[13] concluded that in cases where legal action could result, cell culture should be used for diagnosis of CT. The manufacturers of EIA tests (eg NOVOBIO Ltd) state that the test is unsuitable for specimens contaminated with faeces (including rectal swabs). Micro-immunofluorescence requires further evaluation in children.

Infection in children

The infant may acquire chlamydial infection from its mother during vaginal delivery. The risk of infection appears to be between 50 to 70% of infants born to infected mothers, the major clinical manifestation being neonatal ophthalmia.[14] The most frequent site of infection is the nasopharynx. Asymptomatic infection of the vagina and rectum can occur in as many as 15% of infants born to infected women.[15]

The persistence of CT beyond infancy is controversial. The possibility of persistent perinatally acquired recto-vaginal infection has to be considered in the differential diagnosis of sexual abuse. The isolation of CT from a rectal or genital site raises suspicion of abuse, but in infancy it has been shown that CT may remain dormant for several months after birth.[16] The mechanism is obscure, but infection may spread from the respiratory tract. The possibility that perinatally acquired infection may persist for longer than 2 years should be considered in the evaluation of sexual abuse in children.[17] If a positive *Chlamydia* culture is obtained from a child suspected of abuse, the evidence for abuse is strengthened if asymptomatic maternal infection has been excluded and urethral infection in the alleged perpetrator can be demonstrated by culture.

Rectogenital CT infection was identified in 4 to 17% of sexually abused children when specimens were routinely cultured.[14,19,53]

CT infection is more common than gonorrhoea in adults. The lower isolation rates in children may be due to low infection rates of the vagina compared with the endocervix.[18] Most girls with vaginal *Chlamydia* infection have no symptoms and in a recent study of 49 sexually abused prepubertal girls the proportion with vaginal discharge was the same in girls with and without chlamydial infection.[19]

From the available data there is no evidence that fomites are important in transmission of genital infection with CT. In addition, recto-vaginal infection may persist for several years either after birth or after sexual contact.

Infection in adolescence

Some of the highest rates of infection with CT have been reported in adolescent populations. In a recent study of STD in adolescents (11–18 years) attending genito-urinary medicine clinics in London and Swansea, *Chlamydia* was isolated in 8.5 and 9.5% of girls respectively.[20]

Clinically the infection is associated with cervical inflammation and muco-purulent cervical discharge but many girls are asymptomatic. CT is found in 45–50% of women with mucopurulent cervicitis[21,22] but in most studies of adolescent girls, objective criteria, such as the number of polymorphs per HPF on a Gram-stained smear of endocervical secretion have not been used. There are as yet no studies of the risk of acquiring CT in sexually abused postpubertal females or postpubertal male victims of homosexual rape.

Warts

Warts are caused by the Human Papilloma Virus (HPV). Recent typing of HPV DNA by molecular hybridisation suggests that HPV are to a large extent site specific. In adults, genital warts are most frequently associated with type 6 and 11, less commonly with types 16, 18 and others.[24] Site specificity is only partial. HPV 6 and 11 occur in laryngeal papillomas in children[25] and types 1 and 2 have been found in perianal warts.

In adults, genital warts are transmitted predominantly through sexual intercourse and have an incubation period of several months.[26] Less is known about anogenital warts in children. Few cases have been recorded with adequate clinical and virological data and there is a lack of information about the epidemiology and routes of transmission in children. By analogy with adults the responsible virus may be sexually transmitted but viruses may be inoculated during delivery if the mother has genital warts and warts may take up to 2 years to appear.[27] Anogenital warts may arise through non-sexual contact[28] or auto-inoculation as described by Fleming[29] in the case of a 5-year-old boy who had an anal wart and a common hand wart both with sequences of HPV type 2.

Anogenital warts can be an indicator of sexual abuse and appropriate tests should be taken to exclude other STD. The simultaneous presence of another STD in a child would make sexual abuse a near certainty.[30]

Typing of HPV would help to evaluate whether the warts were of genital or non-genital origin and clarify the epidemiology of the disease. However, few centres can offer typing facilities at present and its value in providing evidence against perpetrators is doubtful. Specimens may be stored indefinitely (see Appendix 4b).

Genital herpes

Herpetic infection is caused by Herpes Simplex Virus (HSV) types 1 and 2. Both types of virus can cause all the clinical syndromes and although genital herpes has been attributed to type 2, a number of studies have shown HSV1 to be the cause in as many as 52% of cases.[31,32]

The virus is transmitted by close personal contact including mouth to mouth, genital to genital, orogenital and anogenital contact and has an incubation period of 2–20 days. Infection can come from patients with no apparent herpetic lesions in two situations. Some people who have never had clinically apparent herpes shed virus asymptomatically; others with recurrent genital herpes may from time to time have HSV isolated in the absence of lesions. It has been suggested that inanimate objects are a potential source of infection but the possibility of sexual abuse was not assessed in reports prior to 1968 and in some other outbreaks of HSV attributed to spread by fomites,[33] a common source contact may be a more likely explanation. Transmission by inanimate objects requires the inoculation of infected material with a high virus load from a lesion to an appropriate surface, contact with a susceptible individual, deposition onto a mucosal-epidermal surface and some mechanical friction to aid infection, a combination which makes it an unlikely event.[34] The other methods of transmission may be autoinoculation from an oral infection to the genital area[35] but this is a rare event in adults.

A primary genital herpes infection is usually clinically obvious with the presence of vesicular or ulcerated genital lesions which are painful and associated with tender inguinal lymphadenopathy. Systemic symptoms such as fever, malaise and myalgia are frequently associated with primary infection but are unusual with recurrences.

The standard technique for detecting HSV is by virus culture, for which live intact virus is required. Specimens of vesicle fluid obtained from the base of the ulcer by vigorous rubbing of the ulcers with a cotton tipped swab are placed in suitable transport medium such as Hank's balanced salt solution and dealt with as soon as possible. Specimens should be stored at 4°C if a delay of several hours is expected and can be kept for several weeks. The virus may be cultured in a variety of cell types. Typing is not performed routinely and its value in children would be for epidemiological studies rather than against a possible perpetrator in a case of sexual abuse. However, the recent introduction of restriction enzyme technology has opened the way for 'finger printing' of individual strains[36] and this has been used to demonstrate the uniqueness of HSV isolates from different individuals and to document separate isolates from the same individual.[37] If isolates from a child thought to have been abused and those from an alleged perpetrator are shown to be identical by this technique, this would be strong evidence of sexual abuse. Other newer techniques to detect HSV antigens using monoclonal antibodies or polymerase chain reaction on vesicle fluid or cultured virus may offer suitable alternatives in the future.

Serological tests are of little value in diagnosis because of extensive cross reactivity between HSV types. IgM antibody to HSV reflects active herpetic infection, primary or recurrent, and there is a high prevalence of antibodies to HSV in the general population.

It is important that a full screening for STD is carried out in cases of suspected abuse.

Trichomonas vaginalis (TV)

TV is a unicellular flagellate which is pathogenic in human beings, its only natural host. It lives in the genitourinary tract on squamous epithelial cells of the vagina or urethra in women, and the urethra, prostate and beneath the prepuce in uncircumcised males.[38]

TV is identified in a wet preparation of secretions in physiological saline, the range of sensitivity being 42–92% in adult women.[39] It can be cultured on Kupferburg medium, considered by some the best method of detection.

TV is transmitted by sexual intercourse. Non-sexual transmission is theoretically possible. Live TV has been found in urine and semen specimens after several hours exposure to air and the organisms survive for hours on damp towels and clothing used by infected women.[40] However, non-sexual transmission is believed to be a rare event because the organism is so site specific.[41] Isolation of TV may be used as evidence suggestive of sexual contact.

Neonatal transmission may occur at delivery. Approximately 5% of infants become infected with trichomonads during passage through an infected birth canal.[42] The organism may persist for 3–6 weeks in the neonatal vagina due to the effect of maternal oestrogen and can reside in the urinary tract after disappearance from the vagina.

It should be noted that, because TV does not usually survive for long in the alkaline environment of the pre-pubertal vagina, if the infection is found it suggests recent abuse.

Bacterial vaginosis (BV)

This is a polymicrobial infection in which vaginal anaerobes and *Gardnerella vaginalis* (GV) are present in the vagina. It is one of the commonest causes of vaginitis in adults. It is diagnosed by examining vaginal discharge by Gram-stain for clue cells, a vaginal pH greater than 4.5 and production of a fishy odour after addition of 10% KOH to vaginal secretions.

In children, the normal vaginal pH range has not been established and the pH test cannot be used as a diagnostic guide. GV can be grown from a swab of the vaginal introitus in a variety of laboratory media but the growth of colonies may be obscured by heavy growth of other vaginal flora, unless selective media are used. If practical, vaginal washings are more satisfactory for diagnosis.

The role of sexual transmission in the acquisition of bacterial vaginosis (BV) or GV in adults is not well defined. GV is unusual in cultures from virginal women. It can be recovered from the sexual partners of women with GV.

In a study of 31 abused and 23 non-abused prepubertal girls, Hammerschlag[43] identified possible BV in only one non-abused girl and in a possible eight abused children. In 1987, Bartley et al.[44] found GV significantly more often in 137 sexually abused girls (14.6%) compared to controls (4.2%) and GV was more likely to be isolated from children with a history of multiple episodes of sexual abuse.

The presence of BV or isolation of GV is uncommon in healthy non-abused children and may be acquired after sexual abuse. However it should not be considered as strong evidence for abuse.

Syphilis

Abused children may present symptomatically with either primary or secondary syphilis. Early infectious syphilis is now rare in the UK especially in heterosexuals and few cases have been reported in sexually abused children.[45] Positive serological tests have been identified in some abused children.[46,47]

The organism responsible is *Treponema pallidum* and this can be transmitted transplacentally and by sexual contact, either oral,[48] orogenital[49] or genital.

In cases of suspected abuse when syphilis is a risk, venous blood should be taken for syphilis serology immediately and repeated in 3 months. If lesions of primary or secondary syphilis are suspected, dark ground microscopy should be performed on appropriate specimens. Prepubertal children with early infectious syphilis should be presumed to be victims of sexual abuse.[50]

HIV Infection

There are few paediatric cases in the UK and the majority are associated with the receipt of infected blood products in haemophiliacs. In America the majority of infections with HIV in children up to 16 years are acquired from maternal transmission, intravenous drug use or voluntary sexual activity. However transmission through sexual assault is likely to increase[51] and venous blood for HIV antibody testing should theoretically be taken at the time of examination, at 3 months and possibly at 6 months.[52] The blood samples taken at the initial examination may be stored for HIV testing later if symptoms develop. This may be important in relation to Criminal Injuries Compensation. There are serious ethical considerations in testing a child for a potentially fatal disease for which no effective treatment is available. Testing should not be undertaken without appropriate counselling and consideration.

References

Gonorrhoea

1. Whittington WC, Rice RJ, Biddle JW, *et al. Pediatr Infect Dis* 1988; **7**: 3–10.
2. Groothius J, Bischoff MC, Jauregui LE. *Pediatr Infect Dis* 1983; **2**: 99–101.
3. DeJong A. *Sex Transm Dis* 1986; **13**: 123–6.
4. Tilelli Thurek J, Jaffe AC. *N Engl J Med* 1980; **302**: 319–23.
5. White ST, Loda FA, Ingram DL, *et al. Pediatrics* 1983; **72**: 16–21.
6. Gilbaugh JH, Fucha PC. *Engl J Med* 1979; **301**: 91–3.
7. Henning C, Jacobsen L. Extragenital survival of gonococci. Presented at National Convention of Medicine, Stockholm, 1972.
8. Srivastava AC. *J Med Microbiol* 1980; **13**: 593–6.

9. Branch G, Paxton R. *Public Health Rep* 1965; **80**: 347–52.
10. Farrell MK, Billmire E, Shamroy JA, Hammond RN. *Pediatrics* 1981; **67**: 151–3.
11. Neinstein LS, Goldenring J, Carpenter S. *Pediatrics* 1984; **74**: 67–75.

CT

12. Riordan T, Elvis DA, Matthews P, Ratcliffe SF. *J Clin Pathol* 1986; **39**: 1276–7.
13. Hammerschlag MR, Roblin PM, Sanchez N, *et al. Pediatr Res* 1988; **23**: 292A.
14. Hammerschlag MR. *J Pediatr* 1989; **114**(5): 727–34.
15. Schachter J, Grossman M, Sweet RL. *J Am Med Assoc* 1986; **225**: 3374–7.
16. Bell TA, Stamm WE, Knoll, *et al. Pediatr Infect Dis* 1987; **6**: 928–31.
17. Bell TA, Stamm WE. Chlamydial trachomatis infections in infants. 1986; 305–8.
18. Ingram DL, Runyan PK, Collins AD, *et al. Pediatr Infect Dis* 1984; **3**: 100–4.
19. Fuster CD, Neinstein LS. *Pediatrics* 1987; **79**: 235–8.
20. Nicol-Thin R, Whatley JD, Blackwell AL. *Genitourin Med* 1989; **65**: 157–60.
21. Burnham RC, Paavoren J, Stevens CE. *N Engl J Med* 1984; **311**: 1–6.
22. Eager RM, Beach RK, Davidson AJ, Judson FN. *West J Med* 1985; **143**: 37–41.
23. Glaser JB, Hammerschlag MR, McCormack WM. *Rev Infect Dis* 1989; **2**: 246–54.

Warts

24. Gissman L, Boshart M, Durst M, *et al. J Invest Dermatol* 1984; **83**(suppl 1): 26–8.
25. Bennett RS, Powell KR. *Pediatr Infect Dis* 1987; **6**: 229.
26. Oriel JD. *Br J Ven Dis* 1971; **47**: 1–13.
27. DeJong AR, Weis JC, Brent RL. *Am J Dis Child* 1982; **136**: 704–6.
28. Rock B, Naghashfar Z, Barnett N. *et al. Arch Dermatol* 1986; **122**: 1129–32.
29. Fleming K, Venning V, Evans M. *Lancet* 1987; **ii**: 454.
30. Oriel JD. *Br Med J* (Editorial) 1988; **296**: 1484–5.

Herpes

31. Chang TW, Fiumara NJ, Weinstein L. *J Am Med Assoc* 1974; **229**: 544–5.
32. Mindel A, Kinghorn G, Allason-Jones E. *et al. Lancet* 1987; **i**: 1171–3.
33. Linneman CC, Buckman TG, Light IJ, *et al. Lancet* 1975; **i**: 964–6.
34. Mindel A. Herpes Simplex Virus 1989. Bloomsbury Series in Clinical Science. Chapter 3.
35. Kaplan KM, Fleisher GR, Paradise JE. *Am J Dis Child* 1984; **138**: 872–4.
36. Lonsdale DM. *Lancet* 1979; **i**: 849–52.
37. Mindel A, Sutherland S. *Antimicrob Chemother* 1983; **12**(suppl B): 51–9.

TV

38. Weston TET, Nicol CS. *Br J Ven Dis* 1963; **39**: 251–7.
39. Editorial. *J Am Med Assoc* 1988; **259**: 1230.
40. Catteral RD, Nicol CS. *Br Med J* 1960; **1**: 1177.
41. Rein MF, Muller M, Holmes KK. *et al. Sexually transmitted diseases.* McGraw-Hill, 1984: 525–36.
42. Thomason JL. *Obstet Gynecol* 1989; **74**(3) part 2: 536–41.

BV

43. Hammerschlag M, Cummings M, Doraiswamy B. *Pediatrics* 1985; **75**: 1028.
44. Bartley D, Morgan L, Rimsza M. *Am J Dis Child* 1987; **141**: 1014.

Syphilis and HIV

45. Ginsberg CM. *Pediatr Infect Dis* 1983; **2**: 232–4.
46. White ST, Loda FA, Ingram DL. *et al. Pediatrics* 1983; **72**: 16–21.
47. DeJong A. *Sex Transm Dis* 1986; **13**: 123–6.
48. Robertson DH, McMillan A, Young J. *Syphilis in clinical practice in STD.* Pitman Medical Publishing 1980: 61–71.
49. Lanigan-O'Keeffe FM. *Br J Clin Pract* **31**: 152.
50. Neinstein LS, Goldenring J, Carpenter S. *Pediatrics* 1984; **74**(1): 73.
51. Gellert GA, Duffee MJ. *N Engl J Med* 1989; **321**: 685.
52. Hager AH. Sexual abuse: the pediatrician's role. 1988.
53. Hammerschlag MR, Doraiswamy B, Alexander, ER, *et al. Pediatr Infect Dis* 1984; **3**: 100–4.

APPENDIX 4b

Sexually transmitted disease in child sexual abuse: Guide to specimen taking and diagnosis

---

Infection screen

The routine specimens to be taken are listed below:

Vulva/vagina or penis

1. With plastic loop or cotton tipped swab take a sample and smear it on a microscope slide for Gram-stain and wet mount in saline on a microscopy slide for *Trichomonas vaginalis*.

2. Take further sample and inoculate directly onto gonococcal medium. If 1 and 2 are not available, swab should be transferred to Amies medium and transported to the microbiology laboratory immediately.

3. With a cotton tip swab take a sample from vagina/penis for culture of *Chlamydia trachomatis*. NB Squeeze swab into *Chlamydia* transport medium bottle, then discard swab. If practicable smear a microscope slide for *Chlamydia trachomatis* antigen immunofluorescence (IF) test (eg MicroTrak), see below.

Pharynx and rectum

4. Take swab from both sites and inoculate onto gonococcal medium.

5. Rectum only. Use cotton tip swab to take sample for *Chlamydia* culture as above. NB Chlamydia EIA (eg Boots Celltech IDEIA/NOVOBIO Ltd, Chlamydiazyme, etc) is not suitable for identification of rectal *Chlamydia*. MicroTrak and EIA are non-specific and non-sensitive in prepubertal children, and culture is recognised as the 'gold' standard for diagnosis of *C. trachomatis* and should be used where legal action could result.

Blood

6. A clotted blood sample should be sent for syphilis serology and for storage. This could be used for HIV and Hepatitis B serology. Ideally, a further specimen should be taken after 3 months.

Others, if indicated

7. If any genital, perianal or perineal ulceration is seen, specimens should be taken with a dry cotton tip swab with vigorous pressure and placed in viral transport medium for herpes culture. The specimen can be kept at 4°C for several weeks for analysis at a later stage. If syphilis is suspected, then dark ground microscopy (discuss with Department of Genitourinary Medicine).

Human papilloma virus: DNA typing

8.   **a**   Fresh material. Transfer as soon as possible for analysis.

     b   Snap freeze in liquid nitrogen. Can be kept indefinitely. Transport in dry ice.

     c   Formol-saline. Stored indefinitely at room temperature and cheap but more difficult for laboratories to process samples.

Incubation period of STD and probability of sexual abuse

Key: *possible; **likely; ***almost certain.

Incubation period	Probability of abuse
Common infections:	
Gonorrhoea 3–4 days	** (*** if child > 2 yrs)
Chlamydia 7–14 days	** (*** if child > 3 yrs and organism cultured in plaintiff)
Herpes 2–14 days	**
Trichomonas 1–4 weeks	***
Warts—several months	*
Bacterial vaginosis	*
Rare infections:	
Syphilis—up to 90 days	***
HIV – majority convert within 3 months	* ⎫ exclude
Hepatitis B—up to 3 months	* ⎭ maternal infections